MIND M

Improve Your Life Using Goals and Budgets

(Advanced Techniques That Improve Your
Memory and Learning Efficiency)

Stephen Holst

Published by Sharon Lohan

© **Stephen Holst**

All Rights Reserved

ISBN 978-1-990334-62-7

Legal & Disclaimer

The information contained in this book is not designed to replace or take the place of any form of medicine or professional medical advice. The information in this book has been provided for educational and entertainment purposes only.

The information contained in this book has been compiled from sources deemed reliable, and it is accurate to the best of the Author's knowledge; however, the Author cannot guarantee its accuracy and validity and cannot be held liable for any errors or omissions. Changes are periodically made to this book. You must consult your doctor or get professional medical advice before using any of the suggested remedies, techniques, or information in this book.

Upon using the information contained in this book, you agree to hold harmless the Author from and against any damages, costs, and expenses, including any legal fees potentially resulting from the application of any of the information provided by this guide. This disclaimer applies to any damages or injury caused by the use and application, whether directly or indirectly, of any advice or information presented, whether for breach of contract, tort, negligence, personal injury, criminal intent, or under any other cause of action.

You agree to accept all risks of using the information presented inside this book. You need to consult a professional medical practitioner in order to ensure you are both able and healthy enough to participate in this program.

Table of Contents

INTRODUCTION

A mind map could be useful for learning and communication purposes. It creates awareness of the components that make up a complex situation. A mind map also provides the possible results of specific actions as well as discerns unacknowledged elements or linkages of a problem or situation.

Have you ever tried using mind maps in determining the possible results of your actions? Learning the basics of mapping will guide you in simplifying the challenges and different situations you are likely to face. You will, therefore, get the best outcome ever. You can determine possible consequences to a specific action while uncovering linkages.

Mind mapping is the best option for those who are not gifted with the power to innovatively think. This is possible due to the capability of mind maps to stimulate skills closely associated with imagination, organization, flexibility, and creativity. Mind mapping promotes the four elements of creative thinking, such as the utilization of colors, shapes, dimensions, and unusual elements. Creative thinking enables an individual to respond to

CHAPTER 1: THE CORRECT WAY TO MAKE A MIND MAP

There are a lot of different ways you could make a mind map, but there is a defined set of symbols and a process for creating a mind map which, if you follow, makes the mind map easier for you to understand and something other people can understand.

Before you start you will need some pens and pencils. If you have some colored ones then that will help. These can easily be picked up at a local store for a few dollars. You will also need some paper, the paper needs to be in landscape format, i.e. the longest edge is at the top. This gives you more typical space to draw your mind map in.

In the centre of the piece of paper you want to write the main concept that you are mind-mapping about. This needs to be in the centre so that everything else can relate to it and radiate out from this central point. This visual method is very helpful in assisting you to remember and understand the core concepts.

If you are mind-mapping a seminar, book or revision then you will write out your mind map as you go along and learn. If you are mind-mapping to solve a problem then your mind map will be much more free-form and you will need to write it out without allowing your conscious mind to interfere too much. You basically just draw the mind map without stopping until you have it all down.

You can be as creative as you want with your mind map. Some people prefer to use boxes and words, whereas others like to use colors and pictures for their mind map. This really is a personal preference and depends upon what works best for you. If the former is best for you then use that, but if you prefer the latter, then use that. There is no right or wrong answer; it's a personal preference.

Often an image can work much better because a picture is truly worth a thousand words and opens up your creativity and other associations. Using color here is a good idea too because it stimulates your brain and grabs your attention. Make sure your picture is a good size because you need to be able to see it clearly and have enough room to join other concepts on to it.

Around this central image you need to put the main points you want to cover. These are words that need to be in capital letters as they are very important. They are like the chapters of a book. Connect these to the central image using bold (or colored) curved links, like a branch to the trunk of a tree.

Printing these concepts in capital letters helps the brain to photograph the words, which allows you to recall it better. Try to use just a single word if you can, as it's easier for the brain to memorize that. If you do use more than one word, do not split it on to separate lines because the line break will disconnect the words in your brain.

If you use curved lines to join these words to the central image this gives a visual rhythm to the diagram, making it easier to remember and is more pleasing on the eye. By making these lines thicker, you are denoting them as being more important, which again, is noted in the brain.

Next you add a second level to each branch. These are again words or images that trigger concepts or information. The words are still printed, but you can use lower case rather than joined up writing. Make the connecting lines thinner because they are further from the centre.

Don't worry about finishing one branch before moving on to the next, you are allowing the information to flow naturally.

The smaller words and the smaller lines denote that these are further from the centre and less important.

You can then add a third and even fourth level of information as you see fit. Again, using images is very helpful because these can convey large amounts of information in a small area. If you are artistically challenged, then you can print out or cut out pictures if necessary.

At these levels, allow your brain to jump around as necessary, recording the information that you need to recall later on.

For some of the key points you may want to add boxes around certain words and images to draw your attention to these points and help you to memorize them.

You may want to draw a colored box around a branch of your mind map, with the box tight to the branch. These outlines can create shapes that your mind can interpret as clouds and help you to remember the concepts. You can use the same colors on different branches to show there is a connection between the branches.

Mind maps are meant to be fun to build, so enjoy the process of making one and get creative. The more you personalize your mind map and make it your own, the more powerful and effective it will be for you.

Below you can see a small mind map based on words and getting fit:

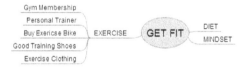

When you draw out your mind map you can expand this, use colors, pictures and more to make a mind map that not only appeals to you but also actually works for you.

CHAPTER 2: WHY MIND MAPPING?

Because the mind jumps from one thing to another, and not in an orderly fashion, linear thinking is extremely limiting. Mind mapping helps you avoid linearly thought processes. A mind map can open your way of thinking in a new and creative direction. Some might say "outside the box." Mind maps are more realistic than lists because like nearly all of life, they are not orderly and ridged to begin with.

Tapping into your right brain hemisphere, where intuition and creativity can be of use, mind mapping encourages problem solving in ways you would not have thought of when using lists and your left, analytical hemisphere of the brain alone. Problems and difficulties are not always going to fit neatly into an outline type arrangement.

Let's say you have 10 things you need to get done today. You take out a slip of lined paper and you list them under the heading

"To Do Today" so you will not forget what to do before you crawl into bed tonight. This is what your list looks like when you're done:

To Do Today

1 - Gas up truck

2 - Lunch with Tony

3 - Email manager

4 - Grocery store for birthday party food

5 - Finish PowerPoint presentation for Thursday

6 - Gym - spinning class

7 - Pay bills TODAY - online

8 - Help Susie with science project

9 - Call client for next meeting date/time

10 - Give Spot a bath

The items on your "To Do Today" list are recorded linearly in a neat numerical and plain layout. Basically, everything you need to complete today is written down; however, there are no colors, pictures or other images to create a more visually stimulating and interesting list.

Using the mind mapping technique, your same "To Do Today" list is laid out in a sprawling style with more space between each item. Then each of the things that need to be done is separated between work and home (or personal and professional if you like). Adding color to the text and connector lines help to engage your right brain hemisphere and so will adding pictures and images.

An example of a mind mapping "To Do Today" style list would have color and pictures to make the list fun and more memorable. For instance, the task "Give Spot a bath" could have a drawing of your dog Spot next to a bathtub following the line that reads "Give Spot a bath". The qualities of the mind map are more dimensional, vivid images and colors help to enhance each of the components.

The idea behind a making a "To Do" list is to have a reminder for the tasks you must complete in a given time frame, in this case, a single day. The written list is problematic from the start for several reasons. For one thing, its construction does not enable easy memorization; it forces review of the list several times during the day. This can also be challenging as it is a time-waster hunting for the list, even if your list is on an electronic device. And if you lose the list, you cannot refer to it and its construction is not meant for your memory; therefore you will most likely forget several of the items needed to be done on your list.

Mind mapping will allow you to create your "To Do Today" list and still use a check-mark system that many individuals find gives them a feeling of accomplishment. Small boxes for checking off "done" tasks can be placed next to each line-item if you wish, and after all, the mind map is your creation, you can fashion it any way that works for you.

A concept map is a diagram in which each parameter contains an idea, concept or problem related by arms to individual.

A concept map seems not always have to be shown as a web but can form as a tree diagram or organisational chart, as an input/output tree or as a flow chart.

Mind mapping is a tool that is distinct from concept mapping. Mind maps have a specific web shape.

Tony Buzan introduced them in the 1970s from psychological theories.

This high-structure idea mapping approach incorporates keywords, photos and colours and is famous for note-taking, brainstorming and creative thinking throughout every generation.

For specific reasons, certain forms of model maps have developed: tree diagrams in organised hierarchical

13

structures, such as hierarchy, input and output trees, for presenting processes.

A mind map is a visual device used to assemble information graphically. It is centralised and represents relations between parts of the entire region.

A mind map typically begins with a single concept, then drawn as an image in the centre of a blank page, where ideologies such as words and pictures added.

Main ideologies are linked directly to the central concept and other subtopics from the core.

Mind maps are close to spider diagrams because their main concepts and sub-ideas set out.

People can make a mental map by hand, for an urgent meeting or lecture, as hard notes; they can also use a specialised pure mapping programme.

Why Is Mapping So Helpful?

For more than 30 years, idea and mind mapping have used in the curriculum for a variety of tasks such as interpreting a definition, taking note and updating.

In reality, a study carried out by the Institute for the Advancement of Education Research, which analysed 29 scientifically-based findings on the use of this technology in schools has shown that they can lead to improved results in several areas, including vocabulary learning, reading and understanding.

Looking at the above list, we find that all areas improved with concept maps also identified as difficult for students with dyslexia, dyspraxia or dyscalculia.

Moreover; Idea mapping can also help manage resources, scheduling, and structure—certain things that might be of interest to those with specific learning disabilities.

Most people with dyslexia enjoy visual imagery and graphically viewing details will improve both imagination and memory.

Images can be used instead of words and features like changing colours; re-sizing and positioning can use to communicate information about the issues, importance or steps to be taken.

Linear research can be organised simply by requiring ideas and concepts to be re-arranged into a diagram conveniently, and concept mapping software can translate into a direct text or display, without thinking about the sentence or grammar form.

Concept maps allow large volumes of knowledge to be graphically processed, making it a useful tool for recall and revision.

You will quickly get an outline of a topic by using keywords on divisions.

Photos and colours may activate emotions, groups or issues.

For additional information, add links leading to archives, sources or websites.

Graphically presenting a concept or problem can help many students to understand links and links to make concept maps a great tool across the curriculum.

Without requiring excellent literacy skills, they are an integrated learning tool for learners of all literacy abilities as concepts and problems can be analysed.

It can be not very easy for people with specific learning disabilities to produce ideas and put them on paper. Concept maps render this task easier: start with a question or template.

Please note ideas, concepts, keywords, processes or images. It forms the map's "nodes." You then add additional thoughts, divisions, to begin building the diagram.

It can also introduce hierarchy into your map, as specific ideas are a subset of others.

It quickly turns into a map.

Why Use Software To Create Mind Maps?

Concept maps have traditionally created with coloured styles on paper.

However, this method provides problems for dyslexic users with bad orthography and handwriting can make it difficult to read a map while organising the plan to fit the paper's limited size.

Furthermore, when a model map to formulate on paper, it can only be used as a guide until done. Ideas can not be re-arranged, extended or changed to another format such as a text version of a map or presentation slides.

You can not confine yourself to an absolute scale with a standard mapping program. You also have access to other instruments, such as pictures and images, spellcheckers and text-to-speech, that help overcome problems and make the map much more usable and presentable.

Hence why so many concept mapping applications also have importing and exporting functionality; information can be converted to a linear, text-based communication format from a visual map (where creators may prefer to work) for communication with others.

Additionally, teachers and support workers may want to build text diagrams then automatically convert them into a design chart that their students may prefer.

For examples, you can import a note text file, then extend and arrange your notes to shape a chart.

Add images and colours to make your notes visually adjustable.

Import the chart to a word processor to a full document or import it to the presentation system to construct a diagram.

Through saving it as an HTML script, you can even build a Web site from your map. You will import activities from Outlook if you are planning a project or want a graphic to - do chart, then create a schedule.

A mind map is an easy and effective graphic visualisation device.

In terms of graphics, mind maps show the connection and structure of concepts in visual form.

By coordination craft, reasoning, and creativity, mind maps help discover the unlimited potential of the human brain.

CHAPTER 4: WHAT IS MIND MAPPING?

A mind map is a diagram used to organize information visually. A brain map is hierarchical and reveals relationships among portions of the entire world. It's frequently created around one idea, drawn as a picture in the middle of a blank page, so that related representations of thoughts such as pictures, words and parts of phrases are included. Important ideas are linked directly to the fundamental idea, along with other thoughts branching out from these significant ideas.

Mind maps are also drawn by hand, equally as "notes" during a lecture, meeting or planning session, as an instance, or as high-quality images when more time can be obtained. Mind maps are regarded as a kind of spider structure.

Much like additional diagramming tools, mind maps may be utilized to create, visualize, construction, and categorize ideas, as well as an aid to analyze and organize data, solve problems, make conclusions, and compose.

Mind maps have lots of programs in private, household, educational, and business situations, such as notetaking, brainstorming (wherein thoughts are placed into the map radially around the middle node, with no implicit prioritization that arrives from sequential or hierarchy agreements, and wherein group and coordinating is earmarked for later phases), outlining, as a mnemonic technique, or to form a complex thought. Mind maps can also be encouraged as a means to collaborate in colour pencil creativity sessions.

Besides those direct usage cases, data recovered from brain maps may be utilized to boost a lot of different programs, such as expert search programs, search engines and research and label query recommender. To accomplish this, mind maps could be analysed with classic procedures of data retrieval to categorize a brain map's writer or files that are linked from inside the brain map.

A mind map is a simple way to brainstorm thoughts without fretting about arrangement and construction. It permits you to structure your thoughts visually to assist with analysis and remember.

A mind map is a diagram for representing jobs, words, theories, or things linked to a fundamental idea or topic with a non-linear graphical design, which makes it possible for the user to construct an intuitive frame around a fundamental idea. A mind map may flip a long collection of dull information into a vibrant, memorable and highly organized diagram that operates in accord with your mind's natural method of doing things.

A mind map may be utilized as a simplified content management system (cms). It lets you keep all of your information in a centralized place to remain organized. With the variety of mind mapping computer software programs available now, you can attach documents to various branches for even more versatility. You can also switch to different various perspectives so as to find one that is best for you. Mind mapping stimulates and challenges you and your staff for brainstorming actions. You will detect some amazing facts about your mind and its purpose and simply take the first significant step on the road to liberty of the brain.

n extremely effective method for getting advice, thoughts, and theories in and outside of your mind -- it is a creative and plausible way of jelqing and note-making that literally 'maps outside' your thoughts.

All mind maps have a few things in common. They've a natural organizational structure that radiates in the middle and uses symbols, lines, colour and graphics based on easy, brain-friendly theories. A brain map converts a long collection of dull information into a vibrant, memorable and extremely organized diagram that operates in accord with your mind's natural way of doing things.

One simple way to comprehend mind mapping would be to compare it to a map of a town. The town centre represents the most important idea; the key streets leading in the centre represent the essential ideas on your thinking process; the secondary streets or branches signify your secondary ideas, and so forth. Particular shapes or images may represent landmarks of curiosity or especially relevant thoughts.

The brain map is the outside mirror of your radiant or natural believing facilitated by a highly effective graphic procedure that offers the universal key to unlock the energetic potential of their mind.

Mind view enables you to think and learn visually by creating mind maps. It's been shown to boost organizational abilities and imagination to create memory retention and deepen comprehension of theories. Not only can it be demonstrated that brain mapping raises learning, memory and thinking abilities, but also the usage of multimedia presentations (incorporating images, videos, sounds etc.) and strongly enhances comprehension and retention of data. Head view is optimized for brain mapping, planning and storyboarding websites and multimedia presentations.

A mind map is a graphic way to represent ideas and theories. It's a visual thinking tool that helps structure info, assisting you to analyze, understand, synthesize, remember and create new ideas. As in every excellent concept, its power lies in its simplicity.

In a mind map, instead of a conventional note or linear text, data is organised in a manner that looks more carefully at how your mind really works. As it's an activity that's both artistic and analytical, it engages your mind in a much richer manner, assisting in all of its cognitive capabilities. And, on top of that, it's fun!

Mind mapping is a kind of visual thinking done by composing one's thoughts in the kind of images or other graphic representation, such as spider diagrams, to get as clear a picture of this topic in question as you can.

It's an employed technique that bridges notions and thoughts. You start by writing down the center idea or thought in the midst of a bit of paper then branch out in all directions together with applicable info and ideas that relate to and create in the first core idea. These associated ideas can then become the cornerstone of additional ideas, and these additional ideas will continue the procedure into fourth grade thoughts and so forth etc.

Possessing a listing on an entire page and then more pages of lists could be a bit daunting and result in confusion; therefore, mind mapping with colors, with an emphasis on words, for example, use of symbols and patterns to help explain thoughts and make inspiration and focus - all of that boosts motivation.

What do you use mind mapping for?

You can use mind mapping for virtually anything, and it'll enable your motivation in many things. Mind mapping is used by psychologists, teachers, engineers and other careers that require intensive believing prior to coming to a finish. It's frequently utilized in business and trade and workplace surroundings. It may be located in training such as brainstorming that are mind maps drawn immediately with flip charts and whiteboards and other websites. It's the thoughts instead of the mind map that are significant in brainstorming. Participation of trainees and workers all add to increase ideas concerning how the true thoughts map may be developed. This exercise can help to reinforce concepts and thoughts more than the usual record ever could!

Additionally, it helps to organise individuals and store info to be able to find out things by remembering the procedure for producing the map particularly. In junior or primary college, mind mapping is introduced into interactive classes that are a lot more stimulating, engaging and inspiring and contribute to kids displaying more excitement in sorting, organising and motivation towards keeping information. Mind mapping can raise kids' purpose and learning capability, and this is especially useful once the child or young person is revising or taking notes in class or in lectures. It's the procedure of creating a mind site in which the learning happens, not the final result.

This is only because you're using one word thoughts or phrases, visual thinking or logos or graphics and graphic representations that have deeper significance for you as well as fit in with the larger image or concept. This helps immensely with memory and remembering that's much more uplifting and inspiring and can lessen the shortage of motivation many frequently experience or connect with revision normally.

Mind mapping is excellent for self-motivation too, so utilize it in your personal life. It can allow you to create and attain significant decisions more quickly and readily.

For example: if you're thinking about beginning a new relationship with somebody, Write the individual's name at the middle of the page and perhaps embellish it with a graphic or graphic representation of a kind that has personal significance for you or draw a circle about it. Then tier from this and then write or draw distinct ideas or concepts that have a relationship with or are a part of this situation with that individual. Maybe you have branches and sub branches that look like symbols or words representing sincerity, enthusiasm, kindness, alluring, beautiful, smart - whatever! Maybe appearing responsible and affectionate, fantastic sense of humor, loves life, considering traveling etc..

Going over your head mapping points later, then you might have the ability to determine adverse or unfavourable traits for deeper thought. So, additional sub branches may include the following theories:

Passionate - constantly occupied with many things, also assertive, rigid, likely to be argumentative.

Has a great job - workaholic, suffers from anxiety, brings home issues from work, no work/life equilibrium.

When you make a mind map and brainstorm matters, writing the first things that come into your mind then looking at it can sometimes describe things straight off by viewing the benefits and pitfalls of any situation immediately. This frequently motivates you to make a decision there and then.

Mind maps cut much of this evaluation that you get from performing lists. Too much research contributes to paralysis, and it is the most frequent illness that slows down advances in several facets of our lives. It may conquer decision making so much with an effect for many that the choice is no more applicable from the time that it's made.

In essence, you're using your intuition and subconscious procedure when doing mind mapping. You're using your five senses to process and report information, not only info in the surroundings, but also information accessible internally from previous knowledge and experiences, which lets you make better choices.

In general, it's a fantastic instrument. Life's problems would not be called "hurdles" if there was not a means to get them over. Accessing and using the power of instinct through mind mapping comes in an awareness of what is occuring in the entire body (felt feeling) in addition to the brain, and this aspect is essential for using your instinct for making better choices, making your revision simpler and more engaging. All this contributes to getting over the barriers, much more motivation, better consciousness and getting things done.

So why is mind mapping deemed to be such a potent instrument. To know why, it's very important to comprehend the idea behind these diagrams. In the event that you should see a brain cell, you'd observe a hexagon such as nucleus with a spindle like branches coming out of it and linking to other cells. Brain cells communicate with each other through those nerve pathways that seem like branches.

So when you're mind mapping, you're mirroring how the brain maps out and communicates its own thought processes. However, there's another significant role and purpose to brain mapping, which is that, if you participate in this procedure, it pushes the ideal side of their mind to talk and speak with the remaining side of their mind.

When you employ this technique, you are plugging a difference that many have, and that's the absence of balance between left and right brain thinking. Most are left brain dominant in how they process information.

The left has to do with the rational and logical processes involved in believing. The right brain consists of the innovative and ingenious thought processes that involve procedures like visualisation, rhythm and instinct like music.

Logic alone informs us that we've been extended a left and right side to the mind with distinct but equally significant contributions to make to the practice of believing, yet the majority of us don't utilize our entire brain.

Mind mapping is one method of assisting to restore this balance, since it promotes lateral thinking where left and right brain need to communicate with each other longer. I find that, if folks try to mind map, at first, it seems somewhat like 'palms and thumbs' since they're forming new patterns of communicating ideas whilst undoing learned customs.

After you write text onto a webpage at the traditional educated form from left to right, that's a linear type of thinking on paper; that isn't how the mind thinks. Studies have demonstrated that people only remember 20 percent of what we read by text independently.

After just a little practice with thought maps, individuals begin to enjoy this process and realize the worth of doing this. It's possible to head map on paper, or it is also possible to use a mind mapping program. Using paper to begin with assists to develop the ability.

However, using applications makes it considerably more potential than direct usage of paper. As an instance, mind mapping software permits you to attach files in one map so you've got them in one area to refer to, rather than having to maintain opening files that are different. Additionally, it lets you web conference and determine different gifts and upgrades to a specific job being worked on, replacing the need to sail to meeting areas to satisfy the identical purpose.

When implemented properly, mind mapping streamlines the process of company growth and personal advancement, thus saving time in addition to increasing productivity, creativity, and learning functionality.

Part of the achievement of mind mapping as a learning and thinking tool is that its use of colour and graphics excite the brain whilst the arrangement of branches mirrors how the brain stores its own memories. It's this that can help us operate through a procedure to embed new words to our memory and will produce an extremely beneficial crib sheet to fall back on.

There are additional methods of utilizing linguistic institutions and eccentric wordplay and vizualization to incorporate language, and they have their place, yet this procedure employs the mind map arrangement to classify and organise words.

Think about a subject around which you want to begin learning vocabulary - for the purposes of the guide, we'll look at words linked to a restaurant. Here are the steps you can undergo:

1. List all the words you need to learn.

2. Categorize them in ways that make sense to you (for instance you may have food, food, beverage, folks).

3. Each class becomes a primary branch to your mind map around the central motif of "restaurant".

4. Each term in the class becomes a sub-branch off the class primary branch (have another colour for every single class). So such as knife, spoon and fork would hang the cutlery off a primary branch.

5. Now draw on your mind map with just images to your branches (you do not need to become an artist; a very simple

thumbnail sketch will do as long as it seems remotely like what the term is).

6. Have a copy of the picture only map.

7. On the next variant, compose the applicable word in your new language beside its image.

When you have completed this, you may have two quite similar mind maps - one with only pictures and the exact same one that's annotated in the translation that is written. A vital portion of doing so is that the true process of categorizing and sorting the words and then coordinating the graphics along with translations will soon be an active learning practice that's a lot more powerful than conventional rote learning techniques.

Additionally, you now have a picture mind map to check your recall of this language and image/word variant to test yourself against and work as a point of reference before you do not want it and have become eloquent in that language.

And the most important thing is that the entire thing could have been interesting, a lot more engaging, and no doubt a great deal of fun. There are different methods of using mind mapping for learning a language, yet this manner of utilizing it for language is among my favorites.

What thoughts mapping does is choose these brainstorming ideas as they develop and set them in a pattern that is focused on that subject or issue. So imagine, when you develop with every thought, every truth, each and every bit of information and then you use a brain map, each and every thing is allocated to a department or section of the map. This gives precious relationships and interconnectedness, which you will not have considered.

You physically watch, or can decide, how one idea relates to the other. In brainstorming, a lot of the relationships are not clear or don't reveal the chances they can generate. Head maps supply the cross-fertilization, the evolution of new thoughts, so beneficial in the imaginative process and for greater productivity. They are especially valuable for entrepreneurs when confronted with having to employ a winning business proposition. For students, there is no better method of making up a workable subject for their own essay or term paper.

This is a brain map about -- handily enough -- head mapping itself. It gifts, in a visual manner, the core components and techniques about the best way best to draw thoughts maps. Yes, I understand this might seem a little too cluttered initially, but bear with me: as soon as you break the ingrained habit of linear note taking, you won't return.

Benefits and programs

The advantages of brain mapping and mind maps work. Fundamentally, mind mapping stops dull, linear thinking, running your imagination and ensuring pleasure.

However, what do we use mind maps for?

Note carrying

Brainstorming (independently or in groups)

Problem solving

Assessing and memorization

Planning

Assessing and consolidating information from multiple resources

Presenting information

Gaining insight on complicated subjects

Running your imagination

It is difficult to do justice to the amount of applications mind maps may have -- the reality is they can help explain your thinking about virtually anything in several distinct contexts: personal, household, educational or company. Planning one day or planning your own life, outlining a book, starting a job, creating and planning presentations, composing blog articles - well, you get the idea -- anything, actually.

o bring a mind map

Drawing a mind map is as straightforward as 1-2-3:

Start at the middle of a blank webpage, drawing or writing the thought you wish to develop. I'd recommend that you utilize the page in landscape orientation.

Build the associated subtopics around this fundamental topic, linking each of them into the centre with a lineup.

Duplicate the exact same procedure for those subtopics, creating lower-level subtopics as you see fit, linking all these into the corresponding subtopic.

Some more recommendations:

Utilize colours, symbols and drawings copiously. Be visual as possible, and your mind will thank you. I have met many men and women who do not even attempt this with the excuse they are "not artistic". Do not let this keep you from trying it out! .

Maintain the subject labels as brief as possible, keeping them into one word -- or, even better, to merely a picture. Notably on mind maps, the urge to compose a comprehensive term is tremendous, but constantly search for opportunities to shorten it into one word or figure -- your own thoughts mapwill probably be more successful that way.

Vary text size, colour and orientation . Vary the depth and duration of these lines. Supply as many visual cues as possible to highlight important points. Every little bit helps engage your mind.

CHAPTER 5: WHY USE MIND MAPS

Some of the benefits of mind maps have already been mentioned but there are more than just those

You Will Remember More

The first benefit of mind mapping is that it can increase your retention of the information. There have been studies done which show that after the initial learning curve for mind maps (which is short by the way!) you can increase your retention of information over traditional note taking systems. The main reason this is assumed to happen is that mind maps encourage better encoding. Encoding is the process of imprinting information on the brain and the better this is done in the first place the better the information will stick. By using drawings, color, and the hierarchical system of mind mapping the brain can encode the information more densely than just a bland old ordered list.

You will make new connections

44

The second way that mind mapping is going to help you is with what is known as convergent thinking. Convergent thinking is just a technical term for connecting different ideas. This type of skill is useful in school because it not only helps information stick better but can lead to better critical thinking skills and if you are writing a paper of giving a speech then this type of connection is exactly what the professor is looking for to show that you have really grasped the course material.

Your creative and brainstorming ability will shoot through the roof

On the flip side of the coin, mind mapping can help with divergent thinking. Divergent thinking is the process of taking one idea and generating several new ideas off of this one and then continuing this process until you have tons and tons of ideas. Mind mapping lends itself to this type of thinking because it starts off from the center as one idea and then branches off potentially as far as you can take it. As an example of this, let's say you wanted to figure out ways to get better grades, You might use this as your central theme and then branch off into study drugs, study skill improvement, attending office hours, learning to take better notes, understanding what type of learner you are, starting study sessions, etc... thinking divergently like this might open your mind to new possibilities which you never knew existed before! When thinking about this very question, I used divergent thinking to find a book which taught me that if you go to office hours with a B paper and ask questions for hours (or until your professor kicks you out!) then they will think twice about giving you anything less than an A. For those of you who are wondering the book is The 4 Hour Work Week by Tim Ferris.

Your notes will be condensed (and you will save trees!)

Another reason to learn the skill of mind mapping is to save space and to make your notes more concise. If you are an improving learner you might find yourself filling out journal after journal with notes and find that you just don't have the time to look back over the mountains of paper which you have used over the past few months. Not only does this destroy countless rainforests (shame on you!) but it also is a hassle to have around and go through. This barrier to studying is part of the reason that normal notes fail. When you learn to mind map, an entire week of classes might fit on one sheet of paper and an entire semester or book will fit on only a dozen or so. When I was mind mapping I was able to keep 4 classes worth of notes in one 100 page notebook.

Your notes will be easier and faster to review

Last but definitely not least is that mind mapping is easier and faster to review. The fact that it is easier makes sense based on the last point but in addition to that it is faster because when you are reviewing a mind map all you have to do is review 100 or so words and phrases and understand the connection between them. Compare that to the style of review which most people do which is sitting down with 20+ pages full of notes and reading them start to finish which can take hours. [i]

Steps to Successful Mind Mapping[ii][iii][iv]

Mind mapping is a simple process but there are a few distinct steps which can help you to get the most out of it

The motto which we are going to use when making our mind maps is **keep things natural.** Mind maps mirror the way we think naturally (in a structured, hierarchical way) and that is the reason they are so effective for boosting memory and creativity, we are going to stick on this same trend and make sure that from start to finish our mind maps are congruent with the way we think, learn, and review.)

Step One: Start with a clear central idea and make a doodle of it

The primary key to mind mapping is choosing the right central idea and stating it clearly. There is a part of the brain called the Reticular Activating System or RAS for short, the RAS is responsible for where we focus our attention and is responsible for what we do and do not notice. This is why people who tend to say "Why does this always happen to me??" tend to focus on the negative and find more examples of why life is hard.

Having a clearly stated central theme with an image will help to train your brain to look for all the information it can gather about the topic later on. When I used mind maps in college as soon as I heard what the lecture was about I would doodle for about 5 minutes and create an image which had some emotion in it in the center of my paper which would focus my attention on finding ideas related to this idea. I remember once I was in a Native American studies class and we were talking about the tribes of Washington State, so for the image I drew an outline of Washington with various images of Native Americans in the middle and then colored the whole thing green because Washington is such a verdant and tree covered state. This image conjured up so much emotion in me that just by thinking of it I can still almost see the mind map in my mind's eye.

The same point applies to mind mapping to take notes on a book or even mind mapping to come up with plans for your business or life. Remember this point and even if you are not a great artist (I am terrible!) just do your best and this technique will ease the rest of the process

Step two: Use one word per line

There is a tendency when we first start using mind maps to tend to add phrases, quotes, or whole sentences on each line of the mind map. This is natural because we think in dialogue and full sentences and whenever we are reading a book or listening to a lecture we are looking at full sentences, learning how to dissect these ideas and distill them down to a single word is one of the greatest challenges and benefits to learning how to use a mind map.

Why all this fuss over keeping things to one word? You might be wondering.

There are many reasons to keep each line to just one word but the most important reason is that doing this helps you to build more associations which is the main benefit of mind mapping. When you use only one word to summarize a point then your mind map will have many more lines even if they are shorter. By having more lines we have more ways to make connections and also there is going to be a greater challenge in making all these ideas fit into the structure of the mind map. By rising to this challenge you will find that you understand the topic better

When I first started mind mapping I had a lot of trouble with this point and I would often break the rules and write out interesting ideas or quotes on lines which led my mind maps to really just be normal notes forced into the shape of a mind map. Doing this really held me back because now I just had awkward to read notes which took up more space than normal! Once I kept my notes to one word per line I started to see a huge benefit in how efficient my notes were, they were more concise and I felt like I understood the technique better.

You might be thinking "What do I do with facts and quotes??"

As far as facts go, I consider these one word, a date or a statistic is a small enough piece of information to include on a line without losing anything. I am a big fan of quotes and I think that being able to remember them is a very fun aspect of learning but they have no place in mind maps. What I will do is if I hear a good quote I will flip the page over and write it as a numbered list. This way on the front of the map I can include a circled number next to the line which is most relevant to the quote.

Colors are more stimulating, use lots of colors, you can use them to code as well.

The next point which is very important is to use color in your mind maps. The brain is more stimulated by colors than by black and white so when you start taking notes in Technicolor you might notice them seeming a little more interesting. This is by no means the only use of color in your notes though, I personally use the color of the category to designate what mood I associate with the branch, we will get into this technique deeper in the next chapter but for now just remember to use a few colors on your map and keep an entire branch one color.

CHAPTER 6: ESSENTIALS OF MIND MAPS

A mind map refers to a visual outcome that occurs from a comprehensive brainstorming over a specified problem or situation. It involves writing your ideas in the form of graphical representation or pictures to obtain a vivid picture of the topic or issue in question.

The concepts involved in mind mapping and mind maps have been practiced for several years now. Such concepts include learning, note taking, visual thinking, problem solving and brainstorming. They have been used by engineers, educations, psychologists, and other professions , which involve detailed thinking prior to getting into a conclusion. Mind mapping has been used as a form of creating thinking for many years already. It has first been evident as far as the 3rd century BC. Porphyry of Tyros, a philosopher is said to be the first to apply mind mapping to create ideas that help others learn easier.

Another adopter of mind mapping and brainstorming is Ramaon Llull. He is a Catalan philosopher as well as the author of the first recognizable work in Catalan literature. Leonardo da Vinci is also said to have applied mind mapping during his note taking sessions. Historians claim that Da Vinci is often considered as the most prominent individual who popularized mind mapping.

Traces of mind mapping were discovered by historians long after Da Vinci in the late 1950s. This is the period when network semantics is thought to have been developed. Network semantics is regarded as a theory that guides individuals in developing learning. It was later supported by Ross Quillian as well as Dr. Alan Collins who was then considered to be the initiator of modern mapping. This arose from his heightened commitment in publishing researches concerning learning and graphical thinking. Quillian and Collins were said to shape mind mapping's future as they utilized a sort of a network wherein all concepts and ideas were integrated through links. These links show how a specific object is associated with another. At this point, mind mapping has become very much used in sharing concepts, learning, and other collaborative methods. However, the popularity of mind mapping has been at its peak during the late 1960s through Tony Buzan, a British psychologist. Buzan created a set of rules, which are to be used during the application of mind mapping.

Apart from professional areas, mind mapping is also used in high school, colleges as well as universities. A good number of mind maps are done with the help of mind mapping software which makes the process more simplified. However, there are still a handful of people who prefer handling them on paper. Mind mapping software cuts the time needed to redraw things after making rearrangements and amendments. It simply provides the links based on the inputs and places them in designated areas of mind maps. In addition, mind mapping software is available in web/cloud-based tools or as a stand-alone application . Other mind mapping programs are also available via smartphones, making it easy for individuals to brainstorm anytime and anywhere they want.

The Significance

Most people question the essence in which mind maps can be useful or helpful. Naturally, they are useful whenever brainstorming is required. For instance, you might have experienced having a brilliant idea prior to writing an essay. However, when you tried to write down your idea, you felt like the idea has ran dry. Perhaps you also might have felt that your ideas do not make sense at all.

This often happens when you failed to organize your work properly and created all possible ideas related with such work. Thus, this is where mind maps can be very significant and useful.

In most cases a mind map is often considered to be a central idea that can be split into a number of ideas or themes. It is carried out using markers or colored pencils. These tools often provide guidelines in determining where the ideas come from. Additionally, they aid in reassessing all the ideas. Mind mapping is a method of note taking, which involves diagrams that result as visual aids. Creating mind maps is easy and learning mind mapping is simple. It can simplify your work substantially. When you write your ideas, you use the left side of your brain, which is more analytical than the right side. The left side of the brain is limited when it comes to creative thinking and can only sustain one idea at a time. On the other hand, the right side of your brain is great for mind mapping. This is because it is the visual part of the brain. Thus, using a mind map will help you get the full picture of all ideas on an immediate basis. You will definitely avoid the processes involved in analytical thinking that often allow you to reflect on one idea at a time.

You do not have to be a good or creative writer. Using a mind map in the required manner will help you generate wonderful ideas. A mind map is a significant tool during brainstorming and collaborating images with words, generating wonderful outcomes.

CHAPTER 7: MAKING YOUR OWN IDEA MAP

Now that you have been introduced to what really is idea mapping and its significance in what you are writing about, this chapter emphasizes on the steps of making an idea map which is definitely an important part in your writing process. How will you make a good writing if you don't do idea mapping and how do you even have an idea map if you don't know how to do one? Here are the steps in idea mapping in order for you to make one and definitely a good one towards the end of this book:

1.Write down the topic. First and foremost, write down your main topic and place it on the center. Without a main topic, there is nothing to branch from when it comes to writing down your other ideas. Identify your focus on the writing that you have to do before anything else. Enclose your central topic with a circle, a box or any shape you prefer. Leave enough space around your central idea for your ideas and map to grow. In the case of writing, this can be your Title.

2. Write down key points. After you have placed your main topic on the center of the page, think of the ideas that are related to it. Connect your key points to your central idea. Branch outward in all directions you would like to from the center. You can do this by drawing a line from your central topic and writing down your key topics along this line. You can also draw a line from the central topic and write down your key point at the other end of it and enclose the word with the shape that you would like to use. In the case of writing, this can be your Chapters.

3. Write down your subtopics. After you have written down your central idea and identified your key points related to it, the next thing to do is complete your outline by writing down subtopics related to your key points and you can do it by branching

out more from the key points. In the case of writing, this can be your Subchapters.

4. Revise. When writing your ideas, just keep on writing and do not think if it will be wrong until you've finish your whole map revising your map comes after that. Go back to looking at the bigger picture and try to evaluate what you have made. Organize your ideas and transfer ideas that are not in their proper category or chapter. This is when you think if you are pursuing to write about a specific topic with emphasis or just making it a subtopic. Remove those ideas that you think you do not have to include. Narrow down your key points, prioritizing the ones that need more emphasis on your writing.

At this point, you have learned what idea mapping is, its importance and significance in your writing process. In this chapter in particular, you have learned how to construct your own idea map and there are actually few steps in doing it and it is relatively easy to really do. First you have to write down your main topic or your title, and then branch out chapters from it and then branch out by writing subchapters. After you have freely written your ideas, you start evaluating your map, revising it, and organizing your ideas. For those who are going to write books, creating a mind map for you chapters of subchapters can be of big help because you are going to deal with more ideas and things to write compared to someone who will be writing a short article.

CHAPTER 8: BENEFITS OF MIND MAPPING

How is mind mapping superior to other means of organizing yourthought process?

Let's look in more detail at the benefits of mind mapping instead of outlining or generic note taking. Let's look at the ways you could organize your thought processes and how mind mapping is more beneficial to you than these other methods. We have already mentioned how mind mapping can help with problem solving in work settings, but it is also highly helpful in your ability to learn, to creatively solve problems, to gather data and record data and information and turn raw facts into substantial plans.

Mind mapping will help you see how this piece of data is linked with that piece of information to form a solution to your problem. A list of information, an outline of problems, or a spreadsheet of data will not help you to see those links so that you can solve whatever problem you may be working with. Most importantly, because the mind map lays out the data and information in the same format that our brains do, it is easy for us to remember and quickly bring to bear on whatever problem we are faced with. The information stored in the mind map will be easy to remember, easy to bring back to the forefront of our minds, and easy to review for solutions.

Part of the success of mind mapping is due to its compact nature. While I might use up several pages taking notes at a presentation or minutes in a board meeting, the person using a mind map in the very same situation might only use one side of one piece of paper. Because of this compact information it is easier to make associations between items and generate new ways of thinking about things. If you have a mind map instead of notes, and more information comes up after the fact, you can easily add it into the mind map in a way that makes sense. On the other hand, if you need to add information into your notes you would usually have to add it to the end of the notes, and it is less likely to be associated easily with other information that it fits with, or linked to present a new view of the issue or information.

Here is a list of generic benefits from mind mapping. When we look later at specific problems that mind mapping can solve, we will also look at the benefits it presents in dealing with those issues and problems. Some of the benefits mentioned here may be reiterated there.

· Mind maps are flexible, allowing for manipulation of information, ideas and knowledge. Most traditional ways of storing information are static while the mind map is dynamic.
· Mind maps can increase productivity by about 20 percent over traditional thought organizing processes. There are several independent studies that show this result.
· Mind maps can increase creativity in problem solving by making it easier to see the connections. With most traditional

methods of organizing data and information, you struggle to find the connections because they are not readily apparent.

· Mind maps identify missing data or information in your notes or thought processes. With traditional methods of organizing data, you often do not even know anything is missing.
· Helps you to "think about your thoughts and your thinking." This means looking at your thoughts and ideas from a larger and more abstract view. This allows you to rethink your processes and ideas. Most traditional means of information organizing is linear and does not allow for this big picture view.

· Mind maps allow for "brain dumps." Now you can see your thoughts in a new way and often come up with a new and creative solution to your problems.
· Mind maps are fast ways to get clarity on your data and information. Many users of mind map software have indicated that this is the number one benefit they get

from mind maps. "Mind mapping expert Kyle McFarlin put it this way: "Mind mapping is the fastest way to get clarity on confusing issues, hands down. No other medium allows you to brainstorm about a subject and quickly rearrange topics, like notes on a desk. And with mind mapping, you get to create knowledge centers for important topics you are working on, all in an easy to see, hub-and-spokes format. It can literally convey what used to take hundreds of pages in one visually engaging document."

· Mind maps help make good and better decisions. Because you get a visual record of the problem as well as the possible solutions, the factors in favor of or against each possible solution, all your brainstorming ideas, allows you the opportunity to come to a better decision than you might if you were just reviewing meeting notes. Quite often you will come to that decision quicker than you would with other methods you have previously used to make decisions.
· Mind maps help you to be better

organized. Mind maps are excellent when you are starting a new project, and you want to link all information together in one place. Your mind map can link not only your ideas, but your agendas and assignment lists, your notes and files. Also you can link relevant web pages and team emails with mind mapping software. You can have everything you need for your project in one place, maybe on one page, so there will be no time lost going through files and piles of notes. It is easy to see how this is an advantage over traditional ways of viewing and organizing material.

· Mind maps help you to see the big picture and the smallest details in your information. This is a magnificent benefit when rethinking the problem or trying to see new connections and new solutions. This is something you could never do with the traditional ways of organizing information.

· Mind maps help to prioritize, identify, and keep track of the key tasks in your project   management.

· Mind maps let you use both sides of your

brain at the same time. You use the right side which is visual and creative and the left side which is logical and analytical. All other forms of information organizing are linear in nature and use only the left side of the brain.

· Mind maps help you make infinite associations and create more ideas as well as stimulating the memory.

· Mind maps also need less storage space and take less time to reproduce and file.

· With mind maps you can tell how important an idea is by how close it is to the starting/primary idea. With traditional information gathering and organizing, it is often impossible to tell which ideas are truly important and which might be secondary.

· Every mind map is unique.

So you can see that there are many, many benefits to mind mapping and an abundant number of ways that this form of information organizing is superior to all others.

CHAPTER 9: THE FOUNDATIONS OF MIND MAPPING

Origins

The concept of mapping your thoughts is not new; in fact, it has been around for centuries. The earliest forms of mind maps have been traced back to the greatest Greek philosophers and artists our world has ever known.

In the early 1950's, doctors began creating "Network Semantics" in order to better grasp the way the human mind works. Shortly thereafter in the 1960's, a psychologist named Tony Bunza took the practice to a level that has made it immensely popular today.

Many incorrectly credit Bunza with creating the mind maps, but what he did was set parameters so that people could recreate them.

The fascination began for Bunza as he began to study the human mind in regard to psychology, neurophysiology, Neuron-linguistics, semantics, information, perception, and general sciences.

Tony quickly realized that while computers came with lengthy operating manuals, the human brain is a billion times more powerful than a computer and comes with no manual to figure out how to use it.

This set in motion the need to write down how and why mind mapping is used by the average person. After publishing over twenty books about the human brain, creativity and learning, Tony Buzan is recognized as an expert in this arena.

The limitations of your brain

We often claim that we are right brained or left brained, but the reality is that we use both sides for different purposes. For example, when you write down a key concept or topic, you are automatically using the left side of your brain, which controls language as the left side of the brain is the logical side.

The right side of the brain, however, controls interpretation of colors, images, depth perception, and the imagination. It is often referred to as the creative side.

The struggle we often face is getting the two hemispheres to work together as the mind's natural inclination is to use one side over the other.

Furthermore, it takes work to move items from our short term memory to our long-term memory. If care isn't taken to make sure that the information is retained, our brains 'dump' the information to make room for the next batch of information.

Take a look at the table below. This represents the work of psychologist Dr. Hermann Ebbinghaus. He mapped the rate that we forget things when we don't take the time to commit them to long-range memory.

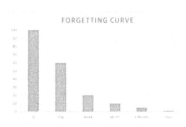

FORGETTING CURVE

At one year, the amount of information retained is nearly zero. Our brains are not designed to store all of the information we are presented with.

These limitation don't need to get in the way of your ability to learn and process knowledge. Our brains are capable of being trained to increase function; it's simply a matter of using the right tools to do so.

2.3 Scientific Connection

Once your mind generates a thought, that thought creates a neuronal path. A neuronal path is similar to a riverbed. When water runs freely through a riverbed, it reduces the chances for that riverbed to dry up and become stagnant, or to eventually disappear.

That's a lot of scientific talk to say that if you repeat an idea often enough, it gets placed in your permanent memory.

For a young child, everything is conscious and requires effort.Actions like walking do not require your conscious thinking anymore because we have done it so often that it has become effortless. Therefore, when you use mind mapping often, you begin to create connections in your brain that did not exist before, which will eventually allow your thinking to become much more effortless as well.

In fact, the total number of connections that can be created by the human brain would total, if laid in a straight line, approximately three miles long.

Our brains are not linear. Our thoughts are free flowing, random, and often jumbled. Furthermore, our thoughts tend to come in the form of pictures. Mind mapping is made to imitate the natural free flowing thinking that takes place in our brains.Mind mapping resonates with our brains because it looks so familiar. Take a look at the image below; this is the glia cell found within the neurons of our brains. Remember this image as it will be important when we show you what a mind map looks like.

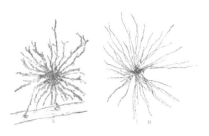

A Mind map looks diagram- which can be color or black and white- and is organized in a way that will help you to develop your thoughts and ideas; the pictures are easily recognized by your brain and require fewer steps in processing.

Scientists have proven that although the two hemispheres of the human brain are identical, they are structured differently (as previously touched on). Many tend to find that they prefer one side to the other and spend more efforts fostering either the right or the left; the best thing you can do, though, is to train the entire brain.

The left side of the brain is responsible for analytical thinking and scientific reasoning, while the right side is responsible for creativity. Mind mapping works to bring out the best of both at the same time.

Mind maps can help you to translate lists of tedious, monotonous information into colorful, highly organized, and easy to remember diagrams that work directly with the brain's natural functions.Since you see a word on paper and immediately visualize the image associated with the word, why not use an image in the first place?

Mind maps draw on the brain's ability to store an infinite number of schemas (connecting new information to old ones) and this, together with their visual qualities (space, image, color etc.) help them to stimulate the memory and recall old schema much faster than linear notes would.

The process can be a pleasurable experience, once you learn all of its particularities and learn to correctly apply it to find solutions for even your most difficult problem.

CHAPTER 10: WHAT IS MIND MAPPING?

Mind Mapping is a form of visual thinking done by writing one's ideas down in the form of pictures or other graphical representation like spider diagrams in order to get as clear a picture of the subject in question as possible.

It is an applied technique that bridges concepts and ideas. You begin by writing down the core thought or idea in the middle of a piece of paper and then branch out in all directions with related information and thoughts which connect to and develop from the original core thought. These related ideas can subsequently become the basis of further ideas and these further ideas can continue the process into fourth tier ideas and so on and so forth.

What can you use Mind Mapping for?

You can apply Mind Mapping to almost anything, and it will help your motivation in most things. Mind Mapping is used by

79

psychologists, educators, engineers and other professions that need intensive thinking before coming to a conclusion. It is often used in business and commerce and office environments. It can be found in training including brainstorming which are Mind Maps that are drawn quickly using flip charts and whiteboards and other media. It is the ideas rather than the Mind Map itself that is important in brainstorming. Participation from the trainees and employees all add to raise ideas as to how the actual mind map might be developed. This exercise helps to strengthen concepts and ideas more solidly. Much more than a list ever could!

It also helps to organise people and store information in order to learn things by recalling the process of creating the map in particular. In primary or junior school - Mind Mapping is introduced in interactive lessons which is far more stimulating, engaging and motivating and leads to children displaying more enthusiasm into sorting, organising and motivation towards retaining information. Mind Mapping can increase children`s motivation and learning ability and this is particularly helpful when the child or young person is revising or when taking notes in class or at lectures. It is the process of creating a Mind Map where the learning occurs not the end result.

This is because you are using one word ideas or phrases, visual thinking or symbols or images and graphical representations that have deeper meaning for you and all fit in with the bigger picture or concept. All this helps enormously with memory and recall which is more uplifting and motivating and can reduce the lack of motivation many often experience and / or associate with revision generally.

Mind Mapping is great for self motivation also, so use it in your personal life. It will help you to make and reach important decisions more quickly and easily.

For Example: If you are considering starting a new relationship with someone.

Write the person`s name down in the centre of the page and maybe embellish it with a symbol or graphical representation of some sort that has personal meaning for you or draw a circle around it. Then tier out from that and write or draw separate ideas or concepts that have a connection with or are part of the situation with that person. Perhaps you have branches and sub branches that appear as words or symbols representing sincerity, passion, kindness, sexy, beautiful, intelligent - whatever! Perhaps appearing responsible and caring, great sense of humour, enjoys life, interested in travel etc.

However, just going over your Mind Mapping points afterwards, you then may be able to identify negative or unfavourable characteristics for deeper consideration. So, further sub branches might include the following concepts:

[Passionate] - always busy with too many things, too assertive, inflexible, inclined to be argumentative.

[Has a Good Job] - workaholic, suffers from stress, brings home problems from work, no work/life balance.

When you create a Mind Map and brainstorm things, writing down the first things that come into your mind and then just looking at it - can sometimes clarify things straight away by seeing the advantages and disadvantages of any given situation quickly. This often motivates you to make a decision there and then.

Mind Maps cut out much of the analysis that you get from doing Lists. Too much analysis leads to paralysis and it's the most common condition that slows down progress in many aspects of our lives. It can prolong decision making so much with a result for many that the decision is no longer relevant by the time it's made.

In essence, you are using your intuition and unconscious process when doing Mind Mapping. You are using your five senses to report and process information, not just information in the environment, but also information available internally from past experiences and knowledge, that allows you to make better decisions for YOU.

All in all, it`s great tool. Life's problems wouldn't be called "hurdles" if there wasn't a way to get over them. Accessing and utilizing the power of intuition through Mind Mapping comes from an awareness of what is happening in the body (felt sense) as well as the mind, and this aspect is vital for using your intuition for making better decisions, making your revision easier and more engaging too. All this leads to getting over the hurdles, more motivation, greater awareness and getting things done.

As the Frenchman Adolphe Monod said; "Between the great things we cannot do and the small things we will not do, the danger is that we shall do nothing".

CHAPTER 11: USING COLORS, SHAPES AND SYMBOLS

The use of colors in your mind map can help you to remember the information that you are mind-mapping. Which colors you use is very much down to personal preference, but there are some colors that almost universally relate to certain concepts:

Green – This signifies go, think about traffic lights here. You can use Green to signify action points.

Red – Often means stop, so can be used for problems or concerns.

Yellow – Can be used for caution or for items that need to be thought about.

Remember that whatever color scheme you choose to use you need to be consistent throughout your mind maps otherwise it is going to get very confusing, very quickly.

You can use shapes for the concepts in your mind map. The recommended shapes vary from expert to expert and between different software programs. Whichever you decide you are going to use, you need to make sure you are consistent in your mind maps.

The main idea at the centre of your page is often illustrated with a circle or oval. If you are using an image, then you can draw a circle or oval around the picture.

You could use a star shape for action points or things to think about. A rectangle can make a good shape to put around your second and third level concepts. You could use a triangle for a concern or problem (remember that many warning road signs are triangles).

If you are using software then you will find that each piece of software will have its own recommended shapes, which can vary.

When drawing a mind map, a lot of people use standard flow chart symbols because it is something that many people learn at school and are familiar with. If you want to use these then that could work very well for you.

Whatever colors, shapes and symbols you decide you are going to use in your mind map, remember that you need to be consistent with them across your mind maps. If you do not remain consistent then you may find that your mind maps become confusing and lose their ability to help you remember things.

Color and shapes are a very powerful way for you to enhance the effectiveness of a mind map. Use them well and you can find your mind maps become easier to remember and far more effective more you.

Chapter 12: Mind Mapping Study Skills

Anyone who is blessed with the gift of sight can easily see the important role it plays in everyday life. Not only do you live within a reality of moving images and pictures, but the most profound thing is that you think and dream in pictures every breathing second. In fact, your entire existence is based on the concept of visual images crisscrossing you like clouds migrating across the sky. With all this in mind, it is no wonder that mind mapping has been considered a fundamental aspect for accelerated learning. We are going to concentrate on the concept of mind mapping in this section and how you can use it for a multitude of reasons in business, at work and at school.

Mind mapping in perspective

Mind mapping is a powerful tool that will help you enhance your ability to learn new information far more effectively and quickly than ever before. This section will cover some applications of mind mapping in detail. You will learn how you can apply mind mapping in a business context, academic circles, and in life. Here are some benefits of mind mapping, and how it affects our everyday actions, decisions, and thinking.

Real life application of mind mapping

The advantages of mind mapping are very dynamic, and actually affect just about every area of your life, helping you grow exponentially and think more effectively due to improved levels of productivity and efficiency to thought.

Provides a universal perspective of information and ideas

A good reason why you find it hard to understand chunks of information is because you fail to view these pieces of information from a global perspective. It is like trying to figure out the earth is round by standing on the ground. If only it was possible to span out of space and look at this piece of information from a universal perspective, we would then be able to see the interconnected chunks interacting with each other in several ways.

Enhances problem solving ability

When you become better at managing and organizing your obstacles within a mind map, you will improve your chances of finding more connections between seemingly defragmented pieces of information. Consequently, this will help you find the answers you might have missed before.

Enhances creative and critical thinking

Your ability to think creatively and critically is based on the foundations of how effectively you can connect seemingly unrelated pieces of information. Using mind mapping can help encourage and enhance the advancement of this type of thinking.

Enhances concentration

Learning or reading information in a linear way tends to put a lot of pressure on your brain. In fact, spending too much time learning this way can become quite draining on your mental resources, and subsequently lead to reduced concentration levels, as well as fatigue.

In most cases, when you read through pieces of linear information, chances are high that you will forget what you've just read because it does not stimulate your mind. On the other hand, mind mapping presents your mind with an exciting stimulus filled with colors, symbols, images, and interconnected pieces that work together to improve concentration and rejuvenate the brain.

Enhances photographic memory

Since you dream, think, and predominantly imagine your world in pictures, it goes without saying that a mind map can help you enhance your photographic memory. For instance, if I tell you to think of a cow... close your eyes and actually think of a cow...

Did you see the word cow in your mind, or did you literally visualize the image of a cow?

Chances are that you saw the image of a cow because this is consistent with how you think about information. A mind map connects and associates words with vibrant symbols, colors, and imaginative images. As far as recalling your mind map from memory is concerned, the written words become secondary, while the visual images, symbols, and color are the ones that leave a lasting sensation on your long-term memory. This works together to help recall information and enhance your photographic memory.

Enhances flow of ideas

When you are able to understand the interactions, connections and associations between different pieces of information, you are able to come up with unique and creative ideas that you would normally not have been able to achieve through ordinary ways of thinking. This is why mind mapping is one of the most powerful brainstorming tools.

Enhances ability to manage information

It's easy to become overwhelmed with the substantial amount of information you are expected to remember and recall these days. It is possible to manage large pieces of information using a mind map. Mind mapping throughout a lecture or seminar will provide you with a sense of confidence and control that will contribute towards your productivity at work, school, and in life.

Enhances confidence

Being able to use mind mapping effectively in the ways mentioned above will naturally improve your confidence, which will help you to effectively manage larger pieces of information.

Career and business applications for mind mapping

Mind mapping can help you enhance your efficiency and effectiveness in the daily management of your career responsibilities and business activities. It will help you clarify your thoughts, save time, and reduce the mental block that you experience when you are bombarded with too much information.

Communicating ideas and message

Mind mapping can come in handy when you are finding it hard to explain a certain idea or concept to a colleague.

Planning time

You can also use mind mapping to better summarize, manage and structure your time based on urgent and important activities. When you have a universal perspective of where you need to concentrate your time, you will be able to feel more in control, and lock in the knowledge that time is completely in your hands.

Planning meeting agenda

Mind mapping can also be used to organize, plan and structure your meetings. Sometimes, you might find yourself a little unprepared in a meeting, and subsequently fail to discuss significant matters. On the other hand, when you use a mind map, you will be able to effectively determine the issues that need to be discussed and addressed throughout the meeting.

Planning company trainings

Mind mapping can also come in handy when organizing and preparing company trainings. When someone is being trained for the first time about certain topics, it can be easy to skip significant pieces of information that the trainees need to understand. On the other hand, when you use a mind map, you will be able to present your knowledge to the recruits more effectively, and help them become better prepared at understanding the ideas from a global perspective.

Planning presentations and speeches

Mind mapping can come in handy in preparing and presenting your presentations and speeches. Sometimes you might forget, skip over, or rush to present vital pieces of your presentations because of a number of reasons. Using a mind map can help you piece your presentation or speech in a focused and structured way.

Planning negotiations

You might find it useful to use mind mapping throughout a negotiation process. If you are negotiating a deal, just put down the details in the form of a mind map, on a piece of paper. This will present you with a universal perspective of the current issues, which will likewise give you unique answers and insights that will help you reach a satisfactory outcome.

Academic applications for mind maps

Mind mapping has been popularly used within academic circles for accelerating recall of information and learning.

As a revision tool

You can use mind mapping as an efficient tool for revising class notes. Since mind mapping provides a global view about a topic, students are able to build strong associations between connected pieces of the subject matter.

For exam preparation

As far as preparing for examination is concerned, there is no better technique to use than mind mapping.

For enhancing memorization of information

Mind mapping tends to mimic your brain's cognitive processes naturally, which makes it a powerful tool for committing large pieces of information to memory. When the information you are studying is in line with your patterns of remembering and thinking, it becomes easy to recall and learn.

For highlighting links and connections

Mind mapping associates, links together and interlocks seemingly unconnected pieces of information in such a way that it makes it easy to recall and remember at a later time. This is why it is one of the most comprehensive tools that can help you gather a global overview and perspective of the subject at hand.

For accelerated learning purposes

Mind maps are very effective in accelerated learning.

Life applications of mind mapping

Daily life management practices and mind mapping don't usually go hand in hand for most people. It's easy to see how it can be applied for career/business and academic purposes, but most people struggle to understand how they can use and implement it in their daily lives. This section will help you overcome some of these misconceptions and provide you with a few guidelines to help you incorporate mind mapping into your everyday undertakings.

As a brainstorming tool

Are you dealing with a problem that needs to be solved? Most people do...

Are you looking for immediate inspiration?

Do you want to know how you can manage an activity or task more effectively?

Just find a piece of paper, have a few crayons and map your ideas and thoughts in a mind map like a child.

To organize lists

Is the long list of things that need to be accomplished overwhelming you?

Do you find yourself panicking at all the things you have to remember to do in the course of your day?

If so, then it might be useful to mind map your tasks on a piece of paper in such a way that you will be able to better structure, arrange and organize them in your mind. Once you have arranged and organized things, you will feel a huge burden lifted from your shoulders. This clarity of thought will improve your memory, as well as your ability to think more efficiently about the activities at hand.

To organize events

Organizing and planning events can exhaust even the most of hardy souls because it can be hard to predict everything that is expected, what must be done at what time, and who must be invited. It can be easy to be overwhelmed and overloaded with all these responsibilities. However, a simple mind map can help you organize, plan and manage your event how you visualized it.

For lifelong quick learning

It is important to understand that mind mapping is not a skill that you learn and use on an occasional basis only. Rather, it is a lifelong commitment that can help you increase the effectiveness and speed of your everyday undertakings.

CHAPTER 13: GROW YOUR MEMORY

WITH THE AID OF MIND MAPPING

The experience will contribute to the memories of many amazing achievements.

Take Mozart's story in 1770, at the age of 14, when he was visiting Rome and listening to the Sixtine Chapel of Allegri's Miserere.

The half-hour piece of music was so rare that the Vatican banned its publishing, but Mozart wrote down the whole piece of music after the performance.

And, more recently, memory champions set world records that seem to ordinary people nothing less than incredible.

These individuals often considered to have incredible intelligence or be incredibly talented. However, in 2002 scientists tested this assumption and conducted several tests on high-ranking memorisers each year at the world memory championships.

The tests showed that the minds of the recall champions display little variations to those of ordinary people.

Nine out of the ten champions in memory discovered, however, to use a technique named' the Loci method,' dating from ancient Greece.

The approach denotes based on place and creativity.

It assumes that a good memory is merely skill and an ability to learn at all times.

The leading theory of memory techniques is to link it with a different concept – it is called a relation.

If your memory has significance, your brain gives a tag that makes it much easier to find.

A similar process is complete when you see something in detail or associated with a different idea that gives the thought a name.

If you think of your memory as a library, finding a specific memory is more comfortable if a tag is attached to it.

You will be surprised how you improve your ability to remember things dramatically by combining association, vibrancy and imagination.

Mind Mapping is the best technique that encourages you to use association and imagination.

Mind Mapping was introduced by Tony Buzan in the 1960s, although some of the greatest thinkers in the world have used and have learned Mind Mapping for hundreds of years.

Tony Buzan says it's the ultimate tool for a thinking-a creative and effective way of thinking which literally' maps out' your brain.

Mind Maps are an ideal tool not only for use as a memory improvement tool but also can have an immediate impact on memory, creativity and your ability to focus.

Mind Maps have a simple form, radiating from the middle, and using a variety of human and brain safe laws, curves, diagrams, terms and pictures.

A long list of repetitive details can be turned into vibrant, unforgettable, highly organised diagrams representing the brain's natural activity and promoting synergistic thinking.

The two main principles that make mind mapping so effective are imagination and association.

You not only improve your ability to come up with innovative ideas by developing creative skills but also by default, increase your ability to remember things.

It is because creativity and memory are vertically identical mental processes—

when you use imagination and partnership, both work best.

1) Recovers all the information you need– your research, an array of coloured styles and a large black piece of paper.

2) Draw a simple picture or symbol in the centre of your page to represent your central idea.

3) Think of the main items or topics of your Mind Map, radiate your key issues as branches to the central image, adding a keyword.

4) Consider now the primary divisions with sub-branches. Attach individual words to each sub-branch. Let your thoughts flow freely and add to each idea a new branch.

5) Use your coloured styles to make your map dynamic and exciting.

6) Alternatively, you can produce your mind map with newly available and exciting mind mapping software, for example.

T only iMindMap of Buzan.

Using software to enable Mind Mapping, it makes it possible for users to produce truly personalised organic Mind Maps, while at the same time incorporating all the principles of Mind Mapping.

Once you have built your Mind Map, you may find that you have one page with all the main points that you need to recall, instead of taking repetitive sequential information.

You will immediately see the connections and connections among different ideas and thoughts.

You can help you gain insight into the grand picture that is the sample on the paper before you.

Second, you used both sides of your brain by creating your Mind Map.

People have a wide range of intellectual and creative skills which they only use in part.

Nevertheless, Mind Mapping profits from the capacity of both the left and the right (creative) sides of the brain.

Therefore, if the right and left brains are related, the two sides are happier and function together to improve their creative output and connection.

It leads to a noticeably improved memory.

CHAPTER 14: WHAT'S A MIND MAP?

The Mind Mapping technique was popularized and brought to the mainstream by British psychology author and educational consultant Tony Buzan.He introduced the use of diagrams to literally and visually "map out" a person's ideas by branching them out. Therefore, instead of the usual format wherein you simply list down your options and ideas, you use a two-dimensional structure that gives a clear picture of the paths that your thoughts and ideas are intended to go.

A Mind Map is in a nutshell, a diagram that is employed to organize information in a visual manner. The diagram is created around a single subject or concept. The diagram usually begins at the center where the subject is drawn.A person creating a Mind Map begins mapping out his ideas from the center of the page.

From there, representations of ideas related and associated with the subject are added. The major ideas are connected to the central idea. From the major ideas, other ideas will branch and so on. This process will eventually create a tree-like diagram. Ideas and thoughts in this diagram can come in various forms. Most common are words, pictures and colors.

Before we go into the details of Mind Mapping techniques, let us take a quick look at its history. Mind Mapping is not a new technique. It has been present among educators, psychologist, engineers, thinkers, writers and researches hundreds of years ago. Some of the earliest traces of these graphical representations of one's ideas and thoughts on paper can be traced to Porphyry of Tyros, a known 3rd century thinker who took the courage to map out visually Aristotle's concepts and teachings.It wasn't until in 1974 however, when Buzan hosted a BBC TV series titled Use Your Head that he introduced to the world the term "mind map".He launched and endorsed the concept and the use of the radial tree.

In a radial tree diagram, key words, which often are colorful and eye-catching, are laid out in a tree-like structure. And like a tree, they allow the ideas to branch out to other ideas. If along the process of mapping out your ideas and other information associated to it, you happen to stumble upon a new idea, you can integrate that into the map with minimal and very subtle disruption of the whole process.

Unlike other forms of traditional outlines and concept maps, Mind Mapping focuses on a single key idea or concept. This allows you to look at the bigger picture and the actual shape of your subject. When you have a bird's eye view of your plans at a single glance, you are able quickly review it and point out any weak links and loopholes.Having a picture in your mind of your plans makes it easier for you to recall its details.

The Mind Map will act as a mnemonic that will commit all the nitty gritty that comes with your plans in your memory. It will become your own memory trigger to help you recall bigger chunks of information and be able to recite them in detail and execute them without needing to go back and review certain documents.Mapping out your thoughts and ideas using pictures, images and colors will not only make Mind Map entertaining. It will also allow them to stand out and attract your attention. Our minds often find it easier to respond to visual representation of things.

A good Mind Map will help you plan effectively by not overwhelming your with details and information. The map should be able to show you the shape of the subject itself, and how the other facts and information relative to it are vital in making your plan or strategy work. And because you can see everything at a glance, you are less likely to forget things, especially those that are crucial to the project's success. It would be easier for you pinpoint where you're at and assess your progress objectively.

Mind Maps can be created in different ways. The most common method is by hand. With a pen and a paper, a person can easily draw and map out his thoughts and ideas. This is commonly used during lectures, meetings and workshops.A more complex diagram can also be created, when a person has enough time on his hands, with pictures and illustrations. Lastly, mind mapping software and programs are now widely available online. These software packages can do more than map out a person's ideas and thoughts. They can also be used to help businesses and big groups organize their operations and processes.

Mind Map is an extremely powerful tool and technique that if used properly, can help unlock the vast and unending potential of the human mind. It can nurture, cultivate and harness various mental skills like spatial awareness and logic. It will develop your skills in using color, numbers, words and imagery in representing your thoughts and ideas. To top all these, mastery of Mind Mapping techniques will give you the freedom to explore you mind. It can propel you to search your mind for more answers and enable it to generate new ideas. Your brain is an unfathomable source of ideas. You just need to know where to look.

CHAPTER 15: FOCUS

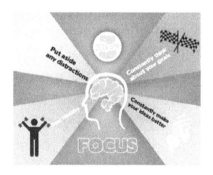

This next step may not require much thought but it is still important to mention since there are a lot of things that can affect the way that we live. These are mostly affected by our surroundings, the people we know, our work environment, where we live, where we hangout etc. Our lives are not completely the same everyday and sometimes the things we experience can set us off track from our goals. This is why you have to make sure that you are prepared for these things.

Tip 1: Put Aside Distractions

I don't even have to explain why having distractions around you will be very detrimental to your progress and how well you are able to organize your thoughts. However, even though none of us want to get distracted from reaching our goals sometimes it is hard to avoid especially if we don't do anything about getting rid of them. It is entirely up to you to deal with this problem. I cannot tell you how to go about it exactly since I do not know what distracts you. However I would still suggest that you try to cut them out of your life if possible.

Tip 2: Constantly Think About Your Goals

Throughout the first part of this book I have constantly reminded you to remember. Constantly thinking about your goals will be helpful in focusing because it reminds you of what you have to do. This in turn will remind you of the ideas and thoughts that you should be putting to good use or should be prioritizing in those certain moments. In addition this has a dual purpose. Aside from the benefit mentioned above you will also be able to achieve your goals faster by thinking about them. You can even find new ways to go about reaching them.

Tip 3: Constantly Develop or Make Your Ideas Better

There is a saying that goes "keep trying until you succeed." Even though it is meant to motivate people I believe that it has negative connotations since doing the same thing again and again until you succeed has a low chance of working and it will only cause stress. I believe that if you fail you have to change your plan and make it better in order to be successful in your next attempt. Constantly developing your ideas will also develop your own critical thinking and will in turn make it easier for you to solve your problems or reach your goals.

Tip 4: Stay Healthy

It is important to keep your body in a healthy state. Why is that? This is because a person is able to do less and think less when he or she is unhealthy or sick. The mind is part of your body and if your body is weak then your mind is weak as well. Without a healthy mind you will not be able to organize your thoughts and ideas more so execute them properly. So the best way to be able to focus is to make sure that you are healthy enough to do it.

CHAPTER 16: HOW CAN MIND MAPS HELP YOU?

In this section you will figure out how psyche guides can support you. A succinct learning strategy will be introduced to you. You will likewise get the opportunity to recognize what your best realizing system is by reflecting upon yourself through the psyche planning measure. At long last, you will be driven through the way toward planning an individual learning plan of your own.

Maybe the most significant thing about psyche maps is that they will permit you to comprehend a subject completely. You are additionally ready to see the most basic components of that point initially. Regardless of whether on a screen or on a bit of paper you can recognize your thought process and what it is that you are attempting to design out. This permits you to conceptualize rapidly and at a more profound level than most different techniques would permit you to do.

Whatever difficult you are attempting to fathom or whatever data you are attempting to comprehend can be handily gotten a handle on when you are utilizing a psyche map. This is the reason mind maps make incredible learning gadgets and are extraordinary for speaking with or showing others too. Since mind maps are so visual, it is anything but difficult to perceive how every subject and theme identifies with each other by how every point is ordered or assembled. More often than not this understanding comes to you initially by the manner in which the data is sorted out.

While you are making a psyche map, you will find that the demonstration itself will assist your thoughts with showing. Basically, as you are contemplating the entirety of the points and subtopics, you will be compelled to make more subtopics so as to push ahead. This, obviously, permits you to break separated the issue or the subtleties of the information considerably further. In the long run, this will give clearness in your reasoning.

The more this data is separated, the snappier you will have the option to comprehend and get a handle on it. At the point when you contrast this cycle with different types of instructive correspondence, for example, in a book, manual, or even an image, you will perceive the amount all the more rapidly the data can be taken in. A psyche map permits you to watch a blend of data in an exceptionally snappy way, making it better than numerous different types of information. One reason why psyche maps are frequently quite a lot more proficient is that you can mix both content and pictures. You can mix the two in any capacity you have to.

Concise Learning Method

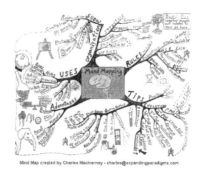

Mind Map created by Charles MacInerney - charles@expandingparadigms.com

The accompanying data was gotten from The Concise Learning Method for 21st Century Students, which was created by Professor Tony Krasnic. The means to this succinct learning technique are as per the following:

Step 1: Preview — The initial step is to see the substance by rapidly looking at the materials previously.

Step 2: Participate — The subsequent advance is to effectively take an interest in a conversation about the material. This will work regardless of whether the conversation happens inside. To do this you could ask yourself inquiries about the subject. This progression starts the commitment which permits you to go from being detached to being dynamic and consequently gainful.

Step 3: Process — In this progression, you consider and store the memory of the point. At the end of the day, this is the point at which your memory of what you have discovered is delivered. This happens naturally when you are making your psyche map. You are intentionally contemplating what you are composing or composing, and this demonstration causes you to envision and recall making this material. As such, recollecting the formation of the brain guide will assist you with recalling the material itself.

Step 4: Practice — When utilizing mind maps, you can 'practice' by composing, re-perusing, or summarizing the material. Discussing the material would likewise assist you with rehearsing. Extremely, any method of auditing the material could be viewed as a 'practice', so don't hesitate to do whatever works best for you. Checking on data multiple times has been appeared to assist individuals with putting away things to memory.

Step 5: Produce — The following stage is to create, or show that you have held the information here and there. This should be possible by composing a report, stepping through an examination, or simply working out what you have gained from memory. This powers you to perceive the data as well as recover it from memory also.

Retention is extremely two unique powers influencing everything. To start with, there is the capacity to perceive data, and second is your capacity to review the data. Recovery of data from memory is a higher ability. It is significant that you're not simply remembering it, that you are really ready to recover it.

The most ideal approach to comprehend this is through various types of testing. Genuine and False or Multiple Choice tests would be instances of tests where you are approached to perceive the correct answer. An Essay Exam, then again, would be a case of a test where you would need to recover the data about a subject from memory. A Short Answer test would be a case of this too. In both condition you are being approached to reproduce the data.

The more that you make the more you'll recollect, yet you should have the option to review the data to make it useable. That is the reason the 'Creation' step is the thing that drives everything home. Reviewing this data and applying it is actually a beneficial demonstration since you are duplicating (or reproducing) the data from memory. Each progression in the process is significant, in any case. Every one of these 5 stages necessitates that you:

Identify key concepts

Meaningfully organize and connect key concepts

Think critically

Ask key questions

You naturally experience every one of these means when you make a psyche map. During the time spent making a brain map you are likewise distinguishing key ideas, interfacing and sorting out those ideas, considering the theme, and posing key inquiries. Accordingly, the demonstration of psyche planning naturally contains the most basic components of this serious learning measure.

Clearly, following this brief learning strategy will assist you with learning and push ahead quicker. Utilizing it all the time through the detailing of psyche guides will duplicate these outcomes exponentially. Tony Krasnic, incidentally, is a firm adherent to utilizing mind guides to speed up learning.

What's Your Learning Strategy?

Presently, move your brain into contemplating the strategies that you can use to learn quicker, retain better, and become more gainful. There are, indeed, an enormous assortment of strategies that you can utilize. They include:

Word ID — Using this strategy includes breaking words into three sections: the prefix, addition, and stem. The prefix can be found toward the start of the word, the postfix can be found toward the end, and the stem is obviously the center of the word itself. Thus, take the word 'submarine' for instance. The prefix of the word, 'sub' signifies beneath and the stem of the word is 'marine', which alludes to water. In this way, by separating the word you realize that a submarine is something that exists underneath water. Having the option to separate words along these lines permits you to more readily comprehend and learn content.

This likewise causes you to show others. You can likewise utilize a brain guide to show this strategy to individuals all the more rapidly. For instance, on the off chance that you needed to show a youngster how to locate the importance of more troublesome words, you could utilize a psyche guide to break words into their segment parts.

Self-Questioning — This strategy includes making questions and afterward searching out the data to answer them. On the off chance that you as of now have the appropriate responses, at that point you can test yourself by posting the inquiries to be replied in the brain guide, and afterward attempting to review them all alone.

Visual Imagery — This strategy includes utilizing mental representation to hold data. For instance, on the off chance that you were heading off to the store to get bread, oranges, and milk, rather than keeping in touch with them out top notch, you could retain them by imagining your outing. In this way, you would envision yourself setting off to the produce segment and selecting the oranges, at that point moving forward to the isle where the bread is at, and afterward moving to the rear of the store, getting the milk and placing it in your crate. In the event that you do this 'stroll through' previously, you will experience no difficulty recalling the things that you need when you get to the store.

This 'stroll through' resembles making a film in your mind. Adding subtleties to your 'film' like thinking about the view or including character will likewise assist you with recollecting subtleties all the more obviously also. For instance, envisioning yourself placing the milk in the crate in your psychological stroll through is presumably going to assist you with recollecting the milk more than any of different items. Presently, if you somehow managed to record these subtleties in a psyche map straightforwardly subsequent to envisioning yourself doing this, this would strengthen the memory you made, making you far less prefer to overlook.

Surmising — The thought here is that you can consider a point and use rationale to reach inferences. At that point, you perform examination to check whether your decisions are right. You can utilize a psyche guide to catch the inquiries, compose them, and afterward attempt to answer them all alone. A while later you go look into the data to locate the genuine answers. At that point, you contrast the appropriate responses that you found and those inside the brain map. You would then be able to add what you figured out how to the brain map, which would drive the learning cycle significantly more.

Quick Paraphrasing & Summarizing — In this technique, you offer short expressions that characterize the subject. As such, when you are picking up something, you can catch the data as short sentences to make the data more important. You can push this technique considerably further by getting watchwords from those short sentences and afterward utilizing a brain guide to make relationship between the catchphrases. You could even get these watchwords from the data that you're considering, and avoid the demonstration of framing the sentences completely. Making the associations between these catchphrases will help you to recover the data from memory, fortifying what you have recently realized.

Paraphrasing — This strategy includes re-composing the data in your own words. Once more, you can strengthen the data by reproducing the data by making a psyche map out of what you summarized.

Reflect

At the point when you think about a specific angles throughout your life, attempt to relate what it intends to you. You can ask yourself what it intends to you corresponding to work, as far as the connections that you have with loved ones, and in the wide feeling of yourself. You're continually learning, so this implies this reflection would change after some time, regardless of whether you need it to or not. Thus, when you experience something new, this offers you the chance to return to a psyche map, reflect again, and update the material.

Changes may happen in an exceptionally brief timeframe. For instance, you may have reflected upon your situation at work, yet then you have a discussion with a colleague which changes your entire recognition. Thus, whenever you open up that brain map, the time has come to reflect again. Another model would be setting off to an instructional meeting or gathering. At the point when you return, you may have a very surprising standpoint about the venture that your business has taken on. Thus, now, you may pull up the old mindmap that relates to that venture, think about what you thought previously, and correct it as per the new viewpoint that you have.

You don't need to play out this appearance before a PC either. You can write down psyche maps on bits of paper anytime. Doing this frequently can assist you with reflecting upon your life, your objectives, and your connections, permitting you to fix your issues, move in the direction of your objectives, and clear your brain on a reliable premise. This would push you to continually soothe pressure, however to persistently be dealing with your objectives also. You can get a great deal out of this, particularly when you consider what a specific subject intends to your life. Set aside the effort to reflect, catch thoughts, and snatch all the open doors that you can to keep the correct standpoint and improve your life.

Design a Personal Learning Plan

The sharpest thing that you can do in your life is to have a procedure made arrangements for learning however much as could be expected. You don't need to record this, yet clearly it is better in the event that you do. Having this system arranged will permit you to apply the perfect strategies at the perfect time. Before you start this cycle, there are a couple of individual inquiries that you should pose to yourself. They are:

For what reason would you say you are realizing what you are realizing?

Would could it be that you are attempting to escape the learning action?

What are you intending to utilize mind planning for?

When would it be a good idea for you to utilize mind planning to get the outcomes that you need?

You are making this arrangement with the goal that you can get the most out psyche planning for your own motivations. You may likewise be doing as such as endeavor to prepare and instruct others. This cycle causes you to find out about yourself and how you learn best, which you can later use to help other people also.

Basically by utilizing mind maps, you can find out about how you learn. You will find out about the sort of language that you use, how you gathering and arrange data, and what best causes you to hold data. Brain planning can assist you with reflecting upon where you have to improve just as where your qualities are.

You can pick the techniques and devices that suit you best and benefit from your time and exertion. Try not to attempt to do it at the same time; it is a learning cycle.

When you have found what your realizing style is, you can apply the learning strategies that work best for you when you are mind planning. Be certain that you utilize a portion of the strategies that have been illustrated above in light of the fact that they are logically demonstrated to work. By figuring out how to utilize mind maps adequately, you can improve your learning, you can all the more likely instruct and train others, and improve your own life, connections, and business.

CHAPTER 17: MAKE A TIMELINE

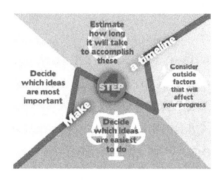

Time is very important to us. There are only 24 hours in one day and that is definitely not nearly enough to be able to accomplish the many things that we want to do. But how is this related to organizing your thoughts? Take this situation for example, you're a college student and a few days from now are your finals. What do you think will be more effective, cramming everything the day before each exam or scheduling and planning out your study time per subject? Making a timeline will also allow you to organize your thoughts in a way that you will be able to focus on the ideas that are needed earlier than the others.

Tip 1: Decide Which Ideas are More Important

Set your priorities straight. Of course the goal is to accomplish everything that you need and want however it cannot be helped that some things will be more important at certain times. So before you make your timeline figure out what things you should focus on more first. For example, in your opinion are your family affairs more important than your work? Are the problems of your friends more important than your own problems? Thinking about these things will help you set your priorities and will help you make a better and more efficient timeline.

Tip 2: Decide Which Ideas are Easiest to Do

Aside from considering importance, it is also important to consider the difficulty of accomplishing the task. Obviously if you put a really hard task before an easy one it will take you more time to finish that task and will possibly set you back a lot. It is important to finish easy tasks first because it helps you build a certain rhythm. It is pretty much the same with writing a book or an essay. The hardest part is getting started but once you have a good start it's all good from then on.

Tip 3: Estimate How Long it will take to Finish Each Task

Not every task will require the same amount of time. Some may take a few minutes, some a few hours or days and some a few weeks or months. This is why it is important to estimate how long each task will take in order for you to create a more or less accurate timeline. You can also look at this as setting a deadline. Setting deadlines helps you learn the discipline and proper work ethic that will foster success in the future. It creates a good kind of time pressure that will help you hone your skills.

Tip 4: Consider Outside Factors that may Affect Your Progress

Not everything will go your way. Luck is always part of the equation as they say and in making an accurate timeline we cannot rely on luck. This is the reason for why we have to make allowances in our schedules or timelines. Everyday random things that change our lives and decisions happen. We cannot predict when and what exactly will happen but we can prepare for the worst. One simple example would be bringing an umbrella when you go out. You never know when it might rain or at least you'll have protection from the sun.

CHAPTER 18: TAKE EFFECTIVE NOTES

" Writing is one thing, and knowing is another. Writing is the photograph of knowledge, but it is not knowledge itself. "
Tierno Bokar (African sage)

The importance of taking notes

The Université québécoise de Laval defines note-taking as "an intellectually efficient and economical way to gather, organize and reduce the information in order to keep only the essentials."

For their part, Bruno Martinet and Yves-Michel Marti recall the following observation in their work on economic intelligence: so-called informal information, that is to say, information that is neither written nor recorded, " represents the major part of information deemed useful by corporate decision-makers. The formalized information represents only a minor part ".

This means that taking notes is an important tool for the manager. Paradoxically, the literature, however abundant on the subject, deals above all with effective note-taking (how to abridge words…) and little effective note-taking.

Who among us, in fact, has never had difficulty in re-reading his own notes, remembering the context that would have given the true meaning of what is written or even capturing a conversation between several people in vain?

And yet we would like it so much:

• Do not lose any important information;

• Easily re-read our notes without having to decipher them;

• Devote more time to listening rather than taking notes;

• Spend less time writing reports, etc.

We will see in this chapter the answer to these expectations, provided by the mind maps, but before, here is an experiment in anticipation of the following: it is simply a question of memorizing all the letters below in one minute. Ready? Go.

D N V E

O S O R

N E R A

N N I P

E S S P

R F E E

U A L L

Is the minute already gone? Well, we will come back to this table of letters soon.

The limits of classic note-taking

In our childhood, we learned to write under the dictation of the schoolmaster, holder of structured knowledge. As adults, many of us continued to implicitly apply this recipe, which did not work too badly in college:

" I now write down everything I can for fear of forgetting, and I will try to understand at home when I learn my lessons. " We can see here that a double effort must be produced:

• capture as much raw information as possible, because of a lack of confidence in our memory (fear of forgetting);

• try to understand our notes, sometimes several hours later, when it comes to exploiting them (who hasn't heard someone admit that they can't read their own words again?).

The heuristic approach

Unlike conventional note-taking, taking notes in the form of a heuristic map (which we will call more simply heuristic notes) first requires us to understand what we perceive in order to be able to write the corresponding keyword or draw the correct image in the card.

First, the consequence of such an inversion (understanding before writing) represents a lesser effort to remember heuristic notes. Indeed, it is easier to remember information that has meaning. For example, if you understood in the previous experiment that you had to read the letters vertically starting from the first column, you probably had no trouble memorizing the sentence "Give meaning to the recall."

Then, by implicitly breaking all connection with time

- ideas are ordered according to our own logic and no longer according to the order induced by the flow of speech or reading - we gain freedom:

• Freedom to note more information, not only the ideas perceived but also the fruit of our own reflection carried out in parallel or even our feelings. In addition, our brain is no longer tempted to filter certain words to maintain a coherent speech heard. It is precisely in the aside or the digressions that an interlocutor delivers, often involuntarily, real treasures of information;

• Freedom to become more critical of the subject matter - We are no longer obliged to follow an argument in the order in which it is presented to us. By reordering the information differently, we have another point of view;

• Freedom to make a perfectly structured and exhaustive synthesis at any time - Ideas are organized in real-time, as and to that extent are written and all fit on one page;

• Freedom to drive or follow the same interview - From a map containing the points to be covered, we can spontaneously complete it or direct the discussion by a question inspired by an empty branch of the map. No more interviews where people have the impression of being "cooked" by an auditor. Make way for semi-structured interviews.

The mind map as a note-taking tool

While it is possible to effectively take notes in the form of mind maps using keywords, this does not necessarily imply obtaining effective notes. Hence the interest in following a method, like the one proposed now and which is inspired by the PERERV method (remember Father Hervé from chapter 1).

Prepare

Just as an athlete gets in condition before a race, taking notes requires physical and mental preparation, even minimal. On the physical side, this consists of checking our equipment (filled pen, OK markers, sharpened colored pencils, etc.) and also installing ourselves in a comfortable place as much as possible.

NOTE - In a meeting, some people routinely sit backlight to see their interlocutor better. Others take care to sit systematically to the left of the person with the strongest decision-making power to better influence him (the importance of this position has been demonstrated scientifically). Without going that far, we must at least pay attention to the ambient clarity so that we can easily re-read our notes.

On the mental side, the preparation varies slightly according to the sources of information (readings, meetings ...), but the idea remains the same: we must put ourselves in a state of questioning in order to be more receptive to the information to which we will be exposed. Don't we say that a person warned is worth two?

NOTE - Who among us has not found, in the days following the purchase of a new car, a sudden increase in the number of identical vehicles on the road: same model and what's more even color. Or did we not see more strollers and newborn babies than usual the day we learned of the arrival of a happy event in our family?

To put yourself in a state of questioning, it suffices ... to ask questions, quite simply:

• What do we already know about the subject (the company that receives me by appointment, the subject of an article or document...)?

• What would we like to learn (during the meeting, thanks to this reading...)?

The answers will help us, in particular, to determine the main branches of the card even before the actual note-taking step.

Once in a state of questioning, we will be like a fisherman who has set down his baits and prepared his lines: we will be able to catch the least important information that passes within reach of our senses. Christian Grellier has a nice formula for summing it up: being prepared also means being "ready to go."

ramify

First good news: knowing how to make cards is implicitly knowing how to take notes effectively. Indeed, taking heuristic notes naturally implies respecting a good part of the advice given in the literature on this subject (extracting the main ideas, practicing active listening, writing legibly...).

No need to try to draw a nice card the first time. Just note as best as possible on a draft sheet the keywords and images as you go because the real structure of the card would only appear clearly at the end.

Second good news: heuristic note-taking is compatible with our work habits. Nothing prevents adding tables, lists, citations, references on the card, for example, in the form of bubbles as suggested by Nancy Margulies in her superb book The organization cards of ideas or via references footer, as in the ordinary text.

read back

Immediately after taking notes, we read the card completely and complete it with information that we did not have time to write. This is especially true during meetings or conferences where memories come back once the tension built up during note-taking is gone.

Let it ripen

" The night is advice," says the proverb. Without waiting that long, it is good to put the map aside for a few moments to do something else, time to let our brain "digest" all the information to which it has just been exposed.

Back home, have we never found the solution to a thorny problem that had taken up a good part of the day at the office, when we didn't even think about it?

Great scientific breakthroughs are often born during breaks after hard work. Thus, Albert Einstein, already cited in the introduction, discovered the theory of relativity restricted by reverie when he imagined himself sitting on a ray of light. August Kekulé understood the ring structure of the benzene molecule while dozing in front of his chimney, while he dreamed of snakes biting their tails. And let's not talk about drowsy Newton and his famous apple…

Reorganize

After the break above, we highlight the important points of our map with color, group together similar ideas with arrows, symbols, add drawings that help us to clarify our notes… In short, we transform the information to better take them over to us.

Perhaps one of the branches is enlarged, a sign that the real subject was not the one announced in the meeting agenda or the title of the article read? Perhaps the presentation of the title, however, so promising, is ultimately uninteresting (spinal map) or, on the contrary richer than expected.

NOTE - This step is very easy when you have a specialized software (see Chapter 8) since reorganization is made directly at the card entry. Concretely, the reorganization can be done at the same time as the cleanup, or in the form of an intermediate map which one builds as one gathers ideas.

Make it clean

We draw in our sketchbook the final map, which will take into account all the modifications made during the reorganization stage. It will thus serve as a starting point for writing a document (classic meeting minutes, memo, etc.), making a decision, etc.

Once the card is finished, we re-read it in order to absorb it fully. This step is particularly useful before speaking in public, and mentally visualizing the map of our speech while speaking gives us great confidence.

This practice is applied to reading texts

We will now apply this approach to the analysis of a text, which can be a simple press article or a large document.

Why work on writing when in the introduction to this chapter, we said that so-called informal information is the most useful for decision-makers? Firstly because the written document is still essential in the business and above all, it is easier to map than a conversation when you start with mind maps.

The preparation

There are many reasons to read a text: by obligation, by need or by desire. In any case, we start. Let's clarify our reading objectives (why read this text) after first reading the text.

A NOTE - To get an idea of the content of an article, read the chapter or the abstract, the titles, the introduction, and the conclusion... For a book, browse the back cover, the table of contents, index looking for interesting keywords, hovering over the start and end of the chapters that caught your attention. Also mark with Post-It ® the passages to be read more carefully later.

Then, we estimate the time allocated according to our own constraints. This will help define our reading strategy (how to read in the allotted time).

Once the objectives have been clarified, we report them in a preparatory map. Then we add to it what we already know about the subject discussed in the text. Thus, our brain will be able to more easily make the connection between our previous knowledge and the information contained in the text.

Finally, we complete this map with what we want to learn from this reading. This last phase puts us in a state of questioning.

Reading

We now put aside the preparatory map which has fulfilled its mission, to read the text in two successive passages:

• a skimming reading intended to identify the main ideas which will be used to build the skeleton of the map ;

• a detailed reading to complete this map with all the information deemed worthy of note.

Skim Reading

We quickly scan the text to find the keywords and the main ideas that we list progressively in the corner of a sheet. These keywords can be known or unknown expressions, which we perceive as important by related to our reading goals and what we want to know.

Then we build a map with this information as the main branches.

Detailed reading

Then we re-read the text in detail and complete the map without worrying about its appearance. The important thing is its content, the real structure of which will only be revealed clearly at the end of the reading.

NOTE - Speed reading techniques can save a lot of time, but unfortunately, they are outside the scope of this book. Consult the bibliography at the end of the book for an example of available methods.

Ripening

Once the reading was over, we deserved a break before moving on to the next phase. And without remorse, thanks to the time savings of 25% consecutive to the questioning and the overview of the text (do not forget that our brain needs time to "digest" the information).

The reorganization

The reorganization is undoubtedly the most interesting phase because it will allow us to distance ourselves from the text and thus perceive the information from a different angle than the author. It is at this moment that the etymology of the word heuristic, that is to say, " which consists or which tends to find, "takes all its meaning.

The cleanup

The cleanup phase does not call for any particular comments since it involves drawing a new map taking into account all the modifications made.

Proofreading

As the PERERV method of Chapter 1 suggests, do not hesitate to contemplate and re-read the finished card. The time spent on this seemingly superfluous activity is actually used to memorize its content. It is also a way to return to the course of an interview or a meeting to analyze cold what happened and complete the map with information initially forgotten.

Trick & tips

Here are some "manufacturing secrets," some of which have been proposed by the community of users of the heuristic map that we already presented in Chapter 1:

• An A4 sheet is generally sufficient to record all the information exchanged during a meeting of two to three hours.

Provide a size A3 for longer durations (seminars, etc.) or when you start with mind maps in order to avoid the "page edge syndrome" (you stop branching out for fear of running out of space);

• To keep a maximum of space during note-taking, a starting rule consists in leaving an angle of 60° between each main branch. As for the secondary branches, the average revolves around three to four ramifications. To position the first branch, just imagine four branches already drawn on the map and start with the highest direction;

• In a sketchbook, draw the map on the right page and the additional notes (tables, citation, bibliographic references...) on the left page (or vice versa depending on preferences) ;

• To practice taking notes in real-time, start by listening to lectures or podcasts available on the internet because it is very easy to modulate the flow rate of the "Pause" button on multimedia players such as Microsoft MediaPlayer or the iPod. Then take notes of telephone meetings because there is no need to take your eyes off the card (it helps at first).

Recommendations

Here are a few recommendations that we often give in training:

• Know how to wait. If you do not know where to attach information to the card, write it, for example, in the corner of the sheet of paper or on a loose sheet. At the end of the 3rd or 4th information, in this case, the common denominator, and therefore the corresponding branch, will appear to you spontaneously, and all that remains is to copy this information into the mind map.

• Persevere. If beginners often find it difficult to take heuristic notes, it is not so much because of the technique itself, much less tiring than conventional note-taking, but rather because it involves an effort of reflection that we are not used to.

• Trust your intuition. Note the first word or draw the image that comes to mind spontaneously. It is necessarily the one who will help you find the information in your memory. Remember, these are just clues to reconnect to your memories.

• Accept mistakes. The fear of "doing wrong" often paralyzes beginners ("is it the right keyword? The right main branch? ..."). Even with more than ten years of practice, we are unable to make a map without erasure during a meeting. In fact, it is even a chance, because the clean up of the card afterward allows us to complete or restructure it. In addition, today there are pens whose gel ink disappears without a trace, under the effect of the heat given off by the friction of the cap on the paper. So, no more hesitation.

In Chapter 9, devoted to the heuristic approach, we will return to the ideas underlying these recommendations, in particular, letting go or even accepting errors.

Value-added heuristic map

Heuristic note-taking makes it possible to perceive information no longer chronologically, as is the case with classical note-taking but in a global and personalized way.

The very technique of mind maps, which requires understanding before writing the keywords, facilitates the structuring of information in real-time as well as its memorization.

This results in a double gain:

• a saving of time in the use of notes (typically, a card reduces by 30 to 50% the time necessary to write a report in everyday language). The gain can even be immediate in the event of an oral summary of a meeting;

• a gain in terms of the quality and quantity of information collected thanks to active listening and better memorization.

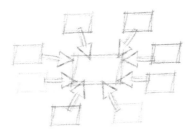

"Teamwork is the ability to work together toward a common vision. The ability to direct individual accomplishments toward organizational objectives. It is the fuel that allows common people to attain uncommon results."– **Andrew Carnegie**

The uses that can be given to Mind Maps are infinite, as many as the imagination and creativity encompass. Next, we will see some examples where they can help to improve different areas.

Educational uses

• Book summaries

You can make summaries of the books that are read in the educational field.

Perhaps the memory comes when a few books have been read, but the situation worsens when many are read or there are books that have been read for a long time and the memory no longer remembers them. In this way, a summary of a book can be saved on a single sheet and have a file with all the books read, which, at first glance, can refresh and strengthen knowledge.

• Study of topics or didactic units

The school textbooks, although they have illustrations, which are erroneously lost as the course progresses, are designed mostly from texts. Carrying out a Mind Map by unit or topic, as a visual summary, favours the understanding of that whole unit completely.

• Brainstorming or brainstorming in group or individual work

When it is necessary to carry out a group or individual work on a subject, as a starting point, a mind map serves to generate a brainstorm that allows an organization of the topics to be discussed and to have an initial photo of the information that will be made up the job.

• Presentation of a group or individual work

For assignments requested by teachers on a particular topic, a Mind Map can be presented as an introduction to the study conducted on the required subject.

It provides a quick synthesis of the work done and helps the maker of said work see if all the necessary points have been covered, as well as the depth of each secondary concept.

• Write an essay

Elaborating a text requires previously thinking about a series of points to be discussed and what better way than through a precious mind map, where the topics to be developed are visualized, with their consequent subtopics and ordered in the most efficient way, for once elaborated, to be able to write all that information in the final writing, without forgetting any point and writing it in a structured and coherent way.

• Other aspects

To delve into a topic, such as writing a book, where the ideas to work, objectives and development of the same are raised.

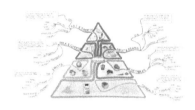

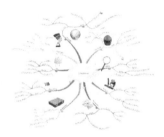

Professional uses

• Launch of a product or service

In the launch of a product or service, there are several key factors that are interrelated, such as the development of the product or service, the commercial direction, the marketing plan, the necessary human resources and the budgets assigned to each area, among others. Many.

See it visually and how they relate to each other, give a picture of the situation, as well as points for improvement.

• Structure of an organization

For the Human Resources department, as well as the management bodies, Mind Mapping can be a great tool for recognizing the current situation of each department and the resources assigned to each of them, both human, economic and material in a single image, to be more effective.

• Short, medium and long term strategic plans

Strategic plans are an arduous work of research, analysis and development, which can be facilitated if you start from a mind map, locating the key points, objectives, resources, etc., ... and from there, develop them.

A Mind Map can also be prepared once all the work is finished as a presentation in a meeting.

• Reorganization of a department

When it comes to reorganizing a department, with a mind map you can visualize in a simple and concrete way the changes to be made, outsourcing, resources, budgets and many more factors that are most likely related and where you can determine which areas gain importance, which must be modified and which can lose specific weight within the department.

•Marketing plan

A marketing plan can originate from a mind map in which to display as notable aspects the objectives to be achieved, the actions to be carried out, the planning of strategies and the public to be reached, for once the critical points have been collected, develop each one of the areas. Once developed, the plan can be presented with the Mind Map

• Other aspects:

Creation of meetings with defined agendas, points of the day to be discussed and objectives to achieve.

Preparation of conferences with schedules, topics to present and key points to highlight.

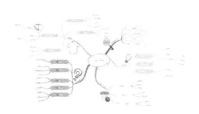

Personal uses

• Your Curriculum Vitae

Present your CV, what an original and creative way! It is sure to stand out among hundreds of CVs. At least yours will surely read or see it. In an increasingly competitive world, you have to use creativity and imagination to be more visible, more recognizable and prominent, and with a mind map, you are sure to stand out from the rest.

• Plan vacations

Let's forget the tedious lists of things to take, do or take into account when we go on vacation. With a Mind Map you will have everything at a glance. It sure helps when you have to organize your suitcase to carry the essentials and not forget anything.

• One year personal project

Who has not made that list of objectives (of those that are never met) for the year on January 1st? One of the biggest reasons that goals set from the first day of the year are almost never met is because we only indicate the goal and vaguely. Let's make a mind map by objective to be achieved, with dates to carry it out, means to be used, specific tasks, etc., ...

• Diet to follow

To be able to eat a diet, it takes a lot of effort and discipline. A Mind Map helps to achieve that goal. It can be used as a weekly planning, where every day we draw elements that are necessary such as food, physical exercise, rest and a reminder of foods or customs to eliminate if we want to achieve the proposed objective.

• Creation of a blog or channel on YouTube

Now it is very common to have a personal blog or YouTube channel, but this requires planning, objectives, periodicity of posts or videos, content, length, a strategy ... and with a Mind Map, all these aspects can be clarified.

• Other aspects:

Plan Christmas gifts for the whole family.

Organize household chores for all members of the family.

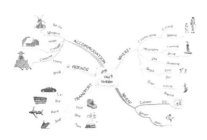

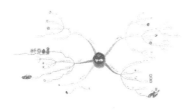

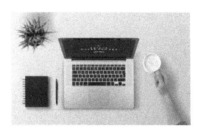

«Man must shape his tools lest they shape him. ». – **Arthur Miller**

Although Tony Buzan recommends drawing Mind Maps by hand, since he considers that the moment in which you draw is essential to think creatively and generate practical ideas, technological tools are also useful, especially if it is an exhibition or presentation on-line.

Thanks to new technologies, there are currently many tools to create Mind Maps, so it will be easy to find the one you like the most or consider the most appropriate.

Next, you will find a list with their respective links to create very attractive and useful Mind Maps for your purposes. They are arranged in alphabetical order and not by importance since, depending on personal tastes and needs, it may vary:

• Ayoa (formerly iMindMap)

The main characteristic of this online tool is that it has the approval of Tony Buzan (as we have already said, the father of Mind Maps). Application that makes it possible to create and personalize Mind Maps promoting creativity, brainstorming and non-linear thinking.

A freemium application with limited content and whose paid version is around € 10 per person. It has an application version to work offline with it compatible with Mac OS and Windows operating systems.

It can be shared with all the members of a work or educational group, allowing everyone to update and modify it at any time. Another great advantage is the ability to attach images, notes and even audio files.

• Bubbl.us

https://bubbl.us/

Software that allows you to create mind and concept maps, without the need to install or download any application. Wide variety of colours, shapes and designs to customize your Mind Maps to your liking.

It can be downloaded as an image and shared with colleagues, collaborators or students. Multi-device tool with which you can work from your computer, tablet or mobile.

• Coggle

https://coggle.it/

Online software to create, develop and share Mind Maps that allows collaboration in real time with any member of the same work group and communication through its integrated chat, to share ideas.

It is a very simple tool to use and it is not necessary to download it, just have a Gmail account to start using it. It allows you to include images, links, share folders, receive notifications in email and has a wide variety of colours, different line formats, branch styles, etc.

It is a freemium tool that allows you to create as many Mind Maps as you want for free, although all of them will be public except for one. For $ 5 per month, you will have the paid version that allows you to have the maps privately.

• CMap Tools

https://cmap.ihmc.us/cmaptools/

Simple tool for developing concept maps. It is completely free and allows you to share the maps created with other people for their realization at the same time.

It can be downloaded on any operating system such as Mac OS, Windows or Linux.

• ConceptDraw

software with a wide variety of forms, images or links. It allows the collaboration of the members of a work group at the same time and can be added to a Power Point presentation.

• Creately

https://creately.com

Freemium application, its free version allows you to create up to five Mind Maps. Great Mind Maps can be created from the web or by downloading the app. Its interface is quite intuitive and allows to develop them easily, allowing collaboration at the same time between students or colleagues.

• EDraw Mindmap

https://www.edrawsoft.com/mindmaster/

This tool has no web version, so it can only be used from the application, which can be downloaded in any operating system such as Mac OS, Windows or Linux. It can be used on the computer or from a mobile device. It has ready-made templates to be able to use them as a base if the user is not yet very familiar with the tool, but it has a wide variety of tools such as backgrounds, objects, symbols, etc.

It can be exported and it even facilitates the uploading of Mind Maps to social networks such as Facebook or Twitter. Ease of inclusion in a Power Point presentation.

It offers special prices for companies, educational institutions and individual students.

• Gliffy

https://www.gliffy.com/

Paid application that has its corresponding free trial period. If the user decides to buy the software after that free period, they can use it from $ 5 per month. Application where all group members can work at the same time and update instantly.

• GoConqr

https://www.goconqr.com/en

Free online tool that can be downloaded and used from a mobile device, in addition to being able to share Mind Maps with the rest of the members of a work or study group and print them. Allows you to attach images for greater versatility of the tool.

Simple-to-use interface, making it easy to start developing Mind Maps in no time and with great results.

• iMindQ

https://www.imindq.com

This online application can be used from the computer through its website for free or desktop version for Windows and Mac OS as well as mobile devices with iOS or Android, these four in paid version.

Like many of the previous ones, files, notes or links can be included and as a distinctive note, it has an integration with

Dropbox to store and save Mind Maps created by users.

• Mapul

https://www.mapul.com

This tool is a web application that allows you to work sharing mind maps with colleagues or collaborators, from a computer, mobile device or tablet.

The freemium version is quite limited and allows you to create a Mind Map, export in jpg and create presentations, when the paid versions, starting at $ 25 per quarter, make it possible to compose unlimited Mind Maps with a greater variety of functionalities, as well as the drawing mode which makes it quite interesting.

• MindGenius

https://www.mindgenius.com/

Tool that only has a 14-day free trial and whose payment plans are higher than the rest because it has access to other types of tools, not just Mind Maps.

It is only usable for the Windows operating system from Windows 7. This tool is simple and very intuitive when working with it.

• MindManager

https://www.mindjet.com/en

Option to get it with a free period of 30 days without having to register your credit card. The paid version for Windows and Mac OS operating systems is expensive (over $ 400).

Despite its price, it is one of the most used tools in the world because not only can beautiful Mind Maps be created, but it also includes other tools, more focused on the business world than on the educational one.

It allows sharing content with collaborators, clients or colleagues on any device, as well as exporting said content to more than 700 web applications.

• MindMapFree

https://www.mindmaps.app/

Free tool with a simple and intuitive interface, without complex menus and with very basic functionalities that allow you to quickly create a Mind Map from scratch. Recommended for individual projects that do not require elaborate and difficult developments.

• MindMaple

https://www.mindmaple.com/

Online tool with a free (and limited) version and a paid version with many more features. As a highlight, to say that it has an option to work with touch screen electronic pen and it is available for Windows ($ 5), Mac OS and iOS ($ 10) operating systems.

It allows you to add notes, links and files to the Mind Map you are creating and export it in different formats such as Word, Excel or Power Point.

• MindMeister

https://www.mindmeister.com/

One of the most popular softwares (more than 7 million users already use it). It has two possibilities, in web format or from the application, although it is not necessary since the web version is quite powerful.

Free (limited to 3 Mind Maps) and with a paid version from € 5. It is designed to be used from Windows, Mac OS or Linux operating systems.

With a great diversity of functions, such as different designs, styles and that makes it possible to attach links and multimedia files, and export them to a presentation.

You can not only generate Mind Maps but also plan projects, create brainstorming sessions. It allows working on a project or Mind Map, sharing and modifying it with the members of a work group.

• MindMup

https://www.mindmup.com/

Although it has a fairly affordable paid version, great mind maps can be made with the free one. It allows you to quickly start making unlimited Mind Maps. In addition, there is the possibility of exporting them in PDF or Power Point and storing them in Google Drive and when creating them, you can attach files, images or icons.

• MindNode

https://mindnode.com/

One of the most popular and free tools for Apple environments, that is, for Mac OS and iOS. Unlimited Mind Maps can be created and it has a wide variety of functionalities, styles and designs, allowing images to be attached and exported in open format, text or image and stored in iCloud. It has a simple and easy to work interface.

• Mindomo

https://www.mindomo.com/it/

Online tool that is in Italian, but if we open it with the Chrome browser, we can use the translator option at the end of the web address bar. It can be used from the computer through its website or download the application to work on it on mobile devices.

With a free version that allows up to 3 Mind Maps and can be shared and published, or paid from € 5.5 where the range of possibilities is expanded such as importing multimedia files or exporting Mind Maps in different formats.

• Mind Vector

http://www.mindvectorweb.com/

Online software for creating Mind Maps, with a simple interface. It has two possibilities, in web format or from the application for mobile devices with iOS or Android operating systems. Its free version (limited to 3 Mind Maps) has quite a few features, although if you want unlimited use of all the tools that the tool provides, you have to get the paid version for $ 9.99.

Mind Maps can be saved to your cloud so they can be accessed by an unlimited number of collaborators, without any problem. It allows attaching files such as images, notes or links, as well as the export of Mind Maps in different formats.

• MindView

https://www.matchware.com/

Tool to create Mind Maps in a very professional way, with a wide range of types of diagrams, maps, templates and other functionalities, which allows you to export files, images or notes in different formats, as well as export them in Microsoft Office environment formats.

Its free version has a trial period of 30 days, the paid versions start from $ 15 per month.

• Popplet

http://popplet.com/

Application that is only in web format (free) or iPad (paid).

With its simple interface, it allows you to quickly start making Mind Maps, allowing you to attach all kinds of multimedia files to your work, creating highly customizable Mind Maps.

• Simplemind

https://simplemind.eu/

Online Mind Mapping tool available for Mac OS, Windows or mobile devices (iOS and Android) in English. Although it has a free version, it is quite limited in features and to be able to enjoy all of them, you have to access the paid versions that start from $ 9.99 for mobile devices.

Images, photos, icons and links can be imported, as well as it is possible to export Mind Maps in image or PDF format. In addition, they can be stored by synchronizing them with cloud solutions such as Dropbox or Google Drive.

• SpiderScribe

https://www.spiderscribe.net/

Online tool that has a free and limited version of public Mind Maps or 3 of a private nature, in addition to three payment plans starting at $ 5 per month, yes, with a 30-day trial period.

Tool focused on Mind Maps and brainstorming whose main feature is the ease of sharing Mind Maps with other collaborators or workgroup colleagues, since it is stored in your cloud and can be accessible from anywhere and on any device.

• The Brain

https://www.thebrain.com/

This free tool has the possibility of being downloaded to the computer's desktop and working from there, online or from mobile devices, with the possibility of accessing the Mind Maps from any of these options.

- WiseMapping

http://www.wisemapping.com/

Software to create Mind Maps without the need to download any application, online and for free. Offers the ability to share Mind Maps, as well as insert them into web pages. With a simple interface and with a great variety of functionalities, images and links can be imported, and Mind Maps can be exported.

- XMind

https://www.xmind.net/

Software with free and paid version (from $ 39.99 / 6 months) with all the functionalities. The free version is enough to make beautiful Mind Maps and share them with the rest of your co-workers. Available for Mac OS, Windows and Linux operating systems, as well as mobile devices and being able to work online with it.

It allows importing image files, notes and links, as well as exporting Mind Maps in Office environment formats and in PDF, it can also be synchronized with Evernote. It is one of the most popular tools, in addition to the possibility of making unlimited Mind Maps from the free version, due to its great design with a great variety of functionalities, image banks and templates. They can be saved in your cloud (XMind Cloud) and be accessible to all members of the workgroup.

CONCLUSION

The mind mapping techniques in a mind map make it a powerful graphics tool that is capable of unlocking the potential of the brain. It can cultivate the full potential of cortical skills such as image, word, logic, number, color, spatial awareness, and rhythm in a single powerful way. Thus, mind mapping provides you the freedom to explore the infinite areas of your brain.

Mind maps can be applied in almost all aspects of life. They can be significantly used to enhance human performance, generate proper thinking capabilities, and improve their learning skills. Using them on a daily basis will guide you in living a more fulfilled, productive, and successful life. Given that your brain does not have set limits in terms of the number of ideas, thoughts, and connections it can make, it translates that there are also no limits to the various ways you can utilize mind maps to aid you in all aspects of your life.

It is inevitable to face challenges in life. However, mind maps can help you deal with or solve these challenges.

CPSIA information can be obtained
at www.ICGtesting.com
Printed in the USA
BVHW060850310522
638499BV00015B/279